Spirit Led

by Marya Tyler

Spirit Led

Copyright © 2019
by Marya Tyler

2nd Edition

ISBN-13: 978-1982095765

ISBN-10: 1982095768

led by the Spirit, Holy Spirit, Holy Spirit leading,
overcoming temptation, lose weight God's way,
walking in the Spirit, end cravings, Bible weight loss

Printed in the United States of America

ACKNOWLEDGEMENTS

Continuous blessings to my husband Kip whose generosity, faithfulness and kindness are a constant reminder of God's love.

Many thanks to my amazing children and children-in-laws for their support. Special thanks to my daughter Esther who awakened my understanding to the centrality of God's love, and who suggested the title on the back cover.

Special thanks to Ruth Benjamin, whose genuine kindness and valuable insight was pivotal to this book; and to Sally Bair, author of *The Nature of God*, for what were prophetic words of encouragement.

My appreciation to Biblehub.com for making it so easy to examine different versions of the Bible.

All thanks and all praise to God the Father and our Lord Jesus Christ — from Whom, by Whom, and through Whom all things exist. Bless the Lord!

thegracegiventome@gmail.com
The author values your comments.

ABOUT THE AUTHOR

I have no qualifications to write a book about being led by the Spirit except the calling of God on my life to do so. Until age 20, I was desperately confused, especially about how to eat—anxious, craving, and ridden with guilt. I knew nothing of the Bible. Willpower was the only thing I knew.   Mind over matter.

Eventually, it became clear willpower wasn't working, so I turned to drugs. My body slithered into anorexia as my spirit gasped for life.   By God's grace, I finally surrendered all to Jesus. An invisible power beckoned me to follow. It took me to the library, and there my hand reached toward a book. As I cracked it open, a Voice resonated through my whole body:

I am the way.

I looked, and there on the page were the same words:

I am the way, the truth, and the life. No one comes to the Father but by Me. *John 14:6*

With no understanding of the Bible or Jesus or salvation, I relied upon this Spirit to continue to lead me.

With the Holy Spirit as my constant guide, I proclaimed Jesus everywhere, gave away most of my possessions, and within a couple weeks went from a sickly 100 pounds to a healthy 135, where I've remained ever since. Now, and for decades, I've had a wonderfully peaceful relationship with food, free from guilt, continually satisfied, and in blessed health. Jesus Christ will do the same for you.

CONTENTS

CHAPTER 1
POWER TO OBEY

Have you ever wished you had someone who could guide you in every decision: telling you exactly what to eat, what to do, where to go, what to say? If you have abandoned your life to Jesus, you already have that Someone—the Holy Spirit of God.

God's children are led by Him.

> **For all who are led by the Spirit of God are sons of God.**   *Romans 8:14 ESV*

The Holy Spirit teaches us everything we need.

> **The Helper, the Holy Spirit, whom the Father will send in my name, He will teach you all things.**   *John 14:26 ESV*

The Holy Spirit is eager to help every one of us in everything we offer to Him. To yield is to obey. To surrender is to triumph!

Expect miracles.

GROWING UP FAT

I know what it's like to always feel fat, guilty for being fat, and obsessed with eating more at the same time.

I owe my parents a great deal of thanks for not letting my weight skyrocket upward, although that was the way I was headed. My mom made sure we had salad and vegetables every evening, and there was always fruit in the house. Mom kept tabs on what I ate and rebuked me for overindulgence...but still I gained weight. A raging lust controlled my body.

And I truly had woe. My shorts were too tight, my underwear felt cramped, my stomach bloated out and my intestines never really emptied. When my friend Wendy wanted to run, I couldn't keep up. When she wanted to climb a tree, I waited at the bottom. I longed to be able to rise above my circumstances, but I was laden with the shame of lust—lust apparent in my lumpy, surplus flesh.

Even as a teenager, I continued to be totally obsessed with eating every available refined carbohydrate, and hiding the results. I was fat, and I tried to cover my shame.

I wore shirts which hung to my knees. I turned whichever way I needed to keep my bottom out of view of people. Turning my behind away from people's view was a rigid rule I followed at all costs, and to be thought acting strangely was preferable to the humiliation I was sure I would face when they saw how truly large my rear end had become. I no longer stood straight, but allowed my fanny to thrust out backward, for in the mirror, at least from the front, that made me look thinner.

If only I had known the love of God, poured out for all flesh through Christ Jesus. But until I was 20 years old, I knew nothing of the Good News of salvation or the Holy Spirit who would become my Counsellor and constant guide. I assumed there was no hope for me, except mind over body, determination over desire. And I knew I was failing at that game.

THE WORD OF GOD (not a bunch of rules)

The leading of the Holy Spirit is always in tune with the Word of God. The Holy Spirit whispers through the New Testament, which is why when you believe the Word of God, you are transformed. Just as all the lepers, demoniacs, blind, sick and desperate people whom Christ met on the road were set free, so we are set free by the power of the Word of God. Listen:

> **My words... are life to those who find them, and healing to all their flesh.** *Prov. 4:20 ESV*

It's a promise. "Healing to all their flesh." So…what do we have to do to be healed?

> **Jesus answered them, "This is the work of God, that you believe in Him whom He has sent."** *John 6:28 ESV*

This is our work. To believe Him and what He has told us. Period. Do that, and all the rest will follow. Without striving. Without so much as lifting a little pinky of self will. In fact, the less you strive in your own strength, the more powerfully God will work for and in you. Our weakness is His strength.

> **My power is made perfect in weakness.** *II Corinthians 2:9 ESV*

You won't find any rules in this book about what to eat and how much. The fact is, all the dietary laws about portion control and not taking seconds and reducing fat or carbs will probably only exacerbate the problem of lust. Think about those rules and their effect on you. Have they brought freedom?

The Lord Jesus said,
Apart from me you can do nothing.
John 15:5

A man might be able to dissolve most of the fat on his body through extreme physical discipline, but he still wouldn't know how to eat. I learned that by personal experience, and my story is woven throughout these pages.

Now, if the New Testament is the Word of God, and it is, we shouldn't think we can read it any old way. The Word you hold in your hand when you hold a New Testament is God-waiting-to-talk-to-you. Let His Spirit lead you exactly where to read, and listen for His voice whispering what you need to hear at the precise moment.

The Word of God changes our desires. Through faith in It we come to recognize the Holy Spirit's gentle whisper wooing us: "This is the way. Walk in it."

WALKING BY THE SPIRIT

Faith. It moves mountains.

> **Without faith it is impossible to please God.**
> *Hebrews 11:6*

Overcoming an eating problem, like moving any sort of mountain, requires faith. There is no problem too big, even if all you have is a tiny seed of faith.

It's okay to ask God for that tiny seed of faith that will heal your body once and for all. Then trust and believe and thank Him for it. Faith is what pleases God.

> **I tell you, whatever you ask in prayer, believe that you have received it, and it will be yours.** *Mark 11:24 ESV*

So we give thanks. Even before we see the answer.

> **With thanksgiving present your requests to God.** *Philippians 4:6 NIV*

And we walk by faith.

> **We walk by faith, not by sight.** *II Cor. 5:7 ESV*

To walk by faith means to admit we are blind, that we don't see the big picture, and then (this is key) allowing ourselves to be led by the One who does—the Holy Spirit.

> **Walk in the Spirit, and ye shall not fulfil the lust of the flesh.** *Galatians 5:16 ESV*

It's true. We won't overeat if we walk in the Spirit. We won't be greedy if we walk in the Spirit. We won't get caught up in sensuality if we walk in the Spirit. Ask God to carve this verse on your heart.

But what exactly does it mean to walk in the Spirit? As Abraham laid his son Isaac on the altar, so we give our bodies as a living sacrifice to God.

> **I appeal to you therefore, brothers, by the mercies of God, to present your bodies as a living sacrifice, holy and acceptable to God, which is your spiritual worship.**
>
> *Romans 12:1 ESV*

This is how we live. We present our bodies as a living sacrifice for Him to do with as He pleases. A body wholly submitted is what pleases God.

Let go of all rights to yourself. Jesus has a much better plan. Instead of rushing headlong in the power of our own strength and might and wisdom, we wait upon the Lord.

We let go of our own initiative. We simply wait on Him. Rest and wait patiently and don't move until His Spirit gives us the urge to move. In this rest, life begins.

But how do we know when the Holy Spirit is giving us the urge to move?

Try it. Free your mind, focus on Christ, and don't move at all if it means taking your eyes off Christ. Keeping your eyes on the eternal, only move as the Spirit nudges you.

Did you feel it? It is the Holy Spirit's leading.

Even if it feels like you are the one doing the leading, because you are fully submitted to the Will of God without any desire of your own, you know that this is the Spirit of God.

With Jesus, we declare:

Not my will, but Yours be done.
Luke 22:42 NIV

This whole journey called life goes so much better when we let Holy Spirit lead, acknowledging God in everything. Eventually this desire to include the Lord in all decision-making will become a heart attitude, rather than a prayer with words. Eventually it will become like breathing, the desire to do His Will everywhere and always in all things.

Ah… the blessings will flow!

EATING FREELY

Ah, how good it is to eat and be thankful, never questioning, "Should I have eaten that?" Yet multitudes of people, many of them Christian, live under condemnation day in and day out, wondering if they should be eating what they are eating, if they should have eaten what they just ate, and why they are always eating more than they should. It's a nightmare for them—as I know too well.

It took a long time for me to believe that Christ actually wants me to walk in freedom.

> For Christ is the end of the law for righteousness to everyone who believes.
>
> *Romans 10:4 ESV*

Christ came to set us free to eat breakfast, lunch, dinner and plenty of snacks without questioning ourselves and doubting ever again.

> Happy is he who does not condemn himself in what he approves. But whoever has doubts is condemned if he eats, because the eating is not from faith.
>
> For whatever does not proceed from faith is sin. Blessed is the one who has no reason to pass judgment on himself for what he approves.
>
> *Romans 14:22 NAS*

The one who condemns is Satan.
And Satan loves diets. What he hates is the freedom offered to us through the Holy Spirit.

When we set our focus on how we look and feel instead of on God, we say in effect to the Holy Spirit, "I don't trust you." We are putting our self and our tiny understanding of our bodies ahead of the wisdom of the One who made us.

The Lord wants us to look good. It is to His Glory that we live in tune with our bodies. He is exalted when we radiate health and give Him the glory.

The Lord is so very beautiful *(Psalm 27:4)*. He is making us into His image, even settling in us the desire to do what is right.

> **For it is God who works in you, both to will and to work for His good pleasure.**
> *Philippians 2:13 ESV*

So the best we can do is get out of His Way. Abandon the effort, and let Him lead.

GOD'S NOT MAD

God is not mad. Your parents may have ridiculed you. Your brother and sister may have teased you viciously. Your peers may have made fun of you. But Jesus is the very embodiment of mercy.

> As a father shows compassion to his children, so the Lord shows compassion to those who fear Him…For He knows our frame; He remembers that we are dust.
>
> *Psalm 103: 9 ESV*

God is not yelling at us. He's not angrily tapping his elbow with his arms crossed on his chest. He's not spying on your eating habits, talking about you behind your back, and ready to pounce on you for over-indulging. God is close at hand, feeling what you feel, wholly understanding your every motive and every thought.

> For God so loved the world, that He gave His only begotten Son, that whoever believes in Him shall not perish, but have eternal life.
>
> *John 3:16 NAS*

What's not to love about a God who would do that?

> He who did not spare his own Son but delivered Him up for us all, how will He not also with Him freely give us all things?
>
> *Romans 8:32 NAS*

Before we can get our lives straight with the bread in our refrigerator, we need to get our lives straight with the Bread of Life. And that is a simple matter of the heart—letting go of self will, allowing God to fill us all in all. Christ is the nourishment our soul craves.

Jesus came for people with problems. *(Mark 2:17)* That is the first and really only requirement to receiving His miraculous cleansing. If you are a person with seemingly unsolvable problems, He can help. He came for sin-sick folks everywhere.

Christ Jesus uplifts you by His Word. Jesus will not rebuke you harshly unless you reject Him willfully. Even then, He continues to woo you back into fellowship with Himself. He draws you back into His arms where He can take the rejection from your mind by showing you His hands, His feet, His side—He has paid the price for you.

The Lord is not the one condemning you. God is not looking at you with disgust. Yahweh is not worried about your eating habits. Our Lord Jesus is the One who says to the sinner caught in the act of bulimia:

> **Neither do I condemn thee. Go and sin no more.**
> *John 8:11 KJV*

And then He enables the sinner to do just that—to go and sin no more.

When the soul feels guilt it may seem there is no remedy, but true spiritual conviction leads us to respond, "Lord,

I am sorry. It is not within me to do right. Thank you for healing me of this condition and making me new." And because we believe, He will! And He does!

Behold, I am making all things new!
Revelation 21:5 ESV

Faith is what God is looking for. He's not looking at how much you ate. God is looking at your heart and mind. He's hoping to see that before, during, and after you eat, you are abiding in Him. That's all. He's just wanting you to be with Him snuggled up close, believing and trusting, in love with Him as He is in love with you.

Jesus's last words on the cross were, **"It is finished!"** (*John 19:30*) and truly it is finished. Those three words resound eternally with hope and forgiveness for the believer. It is finished. The debt is paid. Your salvation has been bought. You belong to Christ. You are a child of God.

You have received the Spirit of adoption as sons, by whom we cry, "Abba! Father!"
Romans 8:15 ESV

Abba!   Papa!   Dada!   Father!

AM I WILLING?

The Holy Spirit is very capable of leading anyone who is willing to be led. That is the only criterion. A willingness to do the will of God. Jesus said:

> Anyone who wants to do the will of God
> will know whether my teaching is from
> God or is merely my own. *John 7:17 NLT*

In the very same way you will know, if you are willing to do the will of God, whether to buy that package of corn puffs on sale today or not. The question is "Am I willing to do God's will?" If not, let me repent immediately, turning all decision-making over to the Lord. He may lead me to buy it. He may not. I am trusting Him to satisfy me. And He will.

God's heart is broken when we refuse to obey and turn to idols.

> I was crushed by their unfaithful heart
> which turned from Me and by their eyes
> which lusted after their idols. *Ez. 6:9 ESV*

Our Holy Lord God is looking for you to crash the idols of food in your life. And you will. With your heart clinging to Him, you will trample the enemy, you will cast down the idols, you will break the chains that have held you captive. You will be free…at last.

GOD IS ON YOUR SIDE

Who will bring a charge against God's elect? God is the one who justifies; who is the one who condemns? Christ Jesus is He who died, yes, rather who was raised... who also intercedes for us. *Rom. 8:33 ESV*

Remember what Jesus said to the woman caught in the act of adultery?

"Has no one condemned you?" She said, "No one, Lord." And Jesus said, "Neither do I." *John 8:10 ESV*

He forgave her instantly. No doubt Jesus recognized a repentant heart in her, a desire to do what is right, a desire to let go of the old life and be saved. That woman caught in the midst of her filth was me. I am eternally grateful to the Lord Jesus that He released me, not only from perpetual food idolatry, but also from the guilt associated with it.

Never feeling guilty. So wonderful! At this point, Satan has pretty much given up trying to make me feel guilty. Why? Because he knows that I know there is no condemnation for those who are in Christ Jesus.

There is therefore now no condemnation to them which are in Christ Jesus, who walk not after the flesh, but after the Spirit. *Romans 8:1 KJV*

Amen Amen Amen.

SATISFACTION GUARANTEED

When we follow Christ, our satisfaction is guaranteed. That's a promise from Scripture.

> **The Lord will guide you continually, and satisfy your desire.** *Isaiah 58:11 ESV*

He will satisfy your mouth and renew your youth.

> **The Lord…satisfies your mouth with good things; so that your youth is renewed like the eagle's.** *Psalm 103:1 KJV*

A satisfied mouth and a renewed youth. Yea, and Amen!

God knows your thoughts. He knows when you have eaten to silence the lonely ache of a childhood gone awry. He knows when food seemed like the only comfort you had ever had. Your loving Heavenly Father knows your heart cry, and infinitely treasures you with the deepest Love, yearning to lead you by His Spirit so that He can bless you inside and out.

> **For He satisfies the longing soul, and the hungry soul He fills with good things.** *Psalms 107:9 ESV*

Whoever hopes in Christ will be continually satisfied.

YEA, BUT….

I hear you saying, "Continually satisfied? How could that be?"

When I first ran into these promises I too wondered. How could a person like me—so wholly unsatisfied, so continuously ill at ease, so obsessed and guilty about food—how could I ever be satisfied? Reading the Scriptures under the guidance of the gentle Holy Spirit, I began to see that maybe my continuous craving was my own fault. Verses like this one:

> **The righteous eat to their hearts' content,
> but the stomach of the wicked goes hungry.**
> *Proverbs 13:25 NIV*

Hmm, I thought. "The righteous eat to their heart's content? I never feel content. What's wrong here?" Then there were verses like this one:

> **Because of your sins…You shall eat, but not be satisfied.**
> Micah 6:13 ESV

Ouch. It would have been easy to be offended and you know at first I was. But gradually it began to seep into my consciousness that this is good news. If my trouble can be solved by repenting, then it means there is an answer. It means there is a solution!

CHAPTER 2
WALK BY THE SPIRIT

Walk by the Spirit, and you will not gratify the desires of the flesh. *Gal. 5:16 ESV*

How can I walk by the Spirit?

All who are led by the Spirit of God are sons of God. *Romans 8:14 ESV*

What does it mean to be led by the Spirit? These verses point to one of the greatest promises in the whole Bible: **The Lord will guide you continually.** *Isaiah 58:11 ESV*

To be led in perfect righteousness and holiness by the all-knowing God—it takes my breath away to think about. The idea remains a mystery to most professing Christians, yet really it is so simple. Every moment, every step, every decision, we are given the option to rein in our own way and be transformed into God's kingdom people, simply by yielding to the Spirit.

Present your bodies as a living sacrifice, holy and acceptable to God, which is your spiritual worship. *Romans 12:1 ESV*

It's as simple as this. Stop what you are doing. Give your eyes, your thoughts...give it all to Jesus. Like Abraham who tied up his son and presented him on the altar before God, we give over our hands, our feet, our eyes, our fingers—in complete submission to the living God.

> **Present yourselves to God ... and your members as instruments of righteousness to God.** *Romans 6:13 NAS*

Take a look at this Scripture again:

> **Walk by the Spirit, and you will not gratify the desires of the flesh.** *Galatians 5:16 ESV*

Look at what it does not say. It does not say, "Do not gratify the desires of the flesh, and you will walk by the Spirit." It does not say, "Get your act together, stop sinning, and you will walk by the Spirit." On the contrary, it tells us to walk by the Spirit, and we will stop sinning.

It does not say, "Stop standing in front of the open freezer eating out of the ice cream container, and then you will walk by the Spirit. No No. It says, "Walk by the Spirit and you will not stand in front of the open freezer eating out of the ice cream container." See why it's called good news?

You can't control yourself and be controlled by the Holy Spirit at the same time. This is a law more basic to your functioning than breathing.

We need Christ, every moment, every swallow, every decision, every thought. We need Christ in full.

If you have never allowed yourself to be led by God, you are in for such a treat! God is SO GOOD! He has the best avenue for you always, and will lead you in paths of pleasantness, paths of peace. *(Proverbs 3:17)*

You will find creative ideas that you never had before. You will accomplish so much more than you had ever thought possible. You will be bold in ways never known to you before. You will love people as you have never loved them before. Your words will be words of the Spirit instead of the flesh. You will feel the Lord's gentle encouragement guiding you.

Let us then abandon ourselves completely to the One who loves us best. Wait upon God, and you will experience the leading, the motivation and the power to do His will—moment by moment, step by step, day by day by day.

HIS YOKE IS EASY

> Come to me, all who labor and are heavy laden, and I will give you rest. Take my yoke upon you, and learn from me, for I am gentle and lowly in heart, and you will find rest for your souls. *Matthew 11:28 ESV*

You, child of God, are yoked together with Christ. So guess who should be doing all the work? Hint: it's not you. The power of the resurrected Christ is at work in us and through us. Let Him do the pulling. All you need to do is trot along.

Each of us carries a weighty load of responsibility and care, not the least of which is the responsibility to care for our own bodies. Well, imagine this burden as a heavy oxen yoke, and it's on your shoulders. This is the yoke, laden with every care and every worry, that makes it so hard for you to get up in the morning. This is the yoke you drag from the bed day after day. These are the cares you drag around the kitchen, drag to the laundry room, drag to the office, drag back home. These are the cares that almost crush you at times and leave you wishing you had never been born. Now see Jesus lifting this heavy yoke.

> For my yoke is easy, and my burden is light. *Matthew 11:30 ESV*

Jesus is telling the absolute truth. His yoke is easy. His burden is really, truly light. Christ is not asking for you to carry your share. He carries it all. One of Satan's favorite lies is a statement that is not in the Bible: "The Lord helps those who help themselves." No! The truth is, the Lord helps those who have come to the realization that they cannot help themselves. The Lord helps those who rely on Christ as all sufficient. And because Christ is all that we need, we do not need will power. This is the best news ever, eh?

It is not through willpower that you can please God. In fact, willpower will only get in the way. How can Christ carry the yoke for you if you are constantly taking it back on your shoulders and trying to do it yourself?

There is no lasting victory through willpower. You've tried that, right? The victory is in Jesus, in complete surrender—not to the forces of this world, but in complete surrender to Jesus. It is in complete surrender to Him that we experience the load lifting from us and the supernatural power of His Grace taking over. Thank you, blessed Savior.

All that is called for is that we keep tucked in by His side, and tuned in to His will. The All-Sufficient Heavenly Father (El Shaddai) will provide the motivation, as well as the moment-by-moment guidance, to do His will.

This is the good news; this is the gospel we preach.

SELF CONTROL VS. GOD-CONTROL

> The fruit of the Spirit is love, joy, peace ... self-control. *Galatians 5:22 ESV*

We know how fruit grows. Good seed, good soil, water, sunshine. You can't manufacture fruit. And you can't manufacture self-control. Trying to be self-controlled is like trying to be loving, trying to be joyful, trying to be peaceful. You might be pretending to be these things, but the real work of creating self-control in you is done by God, as you abide in Him.

> Abide in me, and I in you. As the branch cannot bear fruit by itself, unless it abides in the vine, neither can you, unless you abide in me. *John 15:4 ESV*

Now, it's true that "self-control" sounds a lot like "self-in-control," as if we should be trying our best to do our best in our own strength. But is that what God wants?

Heavens, no. We do not worship a God demanding willpower; we worship the loving Savior who enables and empowers from within. Didn't Jesus say, "Deny yourself"? How can we deny ourselves if self is in control?

The Greek word often translated "self-control" *egkráteia* actually contains no hint of "self." The direct translation is "dominion within." Dominion within. And who should have dominion within? Not self.

The fruits of the Spirit are not achieved by effort. They are far too precious for that. They grow as we abide in Christ, and let the Holy Spirit have dominion within us.

But...isn't God asking us to exercise control over our bodies? Yes, of course He is. Paul said:

> **I discipline my body and keep it under control.**
>
> *I Cor. 9:27 ESV*

Paul disciplined his body to keep it under control of what? His own self will? Health tips he learned at the forum? No. He disciplined his body to keep it under Christ.

Our discipline of the body is only to keep it under the dominion of the Holy Spirit. Our efforts are not to restrict our calorie intake. Our efforts are not to reduce our portion size. Our efforts are not to balance carbohydrates and protein. Our efforts are to stay in complete surrender to Christ—here, and everywhere. That is the purpose of self, and the purpose of willpower. We get to choose. What should we choose?

Jesus. He is the Way, the Truth and the Life. *(John 14:6)* He alone has the recipe for our lives. When our minds are set on Christ, and we are willing to do His Will, we can be confident that He is leading us. It is in this way we gain control over lust. It is through His leading that food loses its power over us.

> **I say, walk by the Spirit, and you will not carry out the desire of the flesh.**
>
> *Galatians 5:16 NAS*

THE WILL GETS IN THE WAY

A man is told not to cross a line in the sand. Before the line was drawn he never thought much about going in that direction, but now he begins wondering what's across that line. He begins imagining what it would be like to cross over when no one is looking. And at some point, he steps across.

Once a line is drawn, the focus of our attention becomes the line. Our whole viewpoint becomes concentrated on the line. What does your flesh want to do? Cross that line, even if it means you're headed out into the barren desert. Laws have that effect.

The same thing happens when you set yourself a standard: "Read the Bible daily for 15 minutes." You think that should be easy enough to obey, but it isn't long before things get in the way and reading the Bible suddenly seems distasteful. Whereas before you used to love meditating on God's Word, when the rule was set in place, reading the Bible just didn't seem appealing any more. That's the problem with rules.

Our inclination is always to cross that line. Some of us are more compliant than others, but eventually all of us will want to break the rule. And the same thing happens when we draw a line on our eating habits—I won't take seconds, I won't eat snacks, whatever. Immediately our gaze turns to those things we can't eat.

Count calories and you will spend your day thinking about how many calories you can consume. As soon as we draw a line for ourselves—eat only this much—we begin to desire more.

God made one simple request—don't eat from that tree. They could eat from all the other trees in the Garden, but from that tree He commanded them not to eat. And that one little law awakened sin in Adam and Eve. As Paul explains:

> I was once alive apart from the law, but when the commandment came, sin came alive and I died. *Romans 7:9 ESV*

The law awakens sin.

SIN CAME ALIVE

AGE 4. It happened to me something like this: I had been invited to the neighbor's house for lunch. They had a child my age, and this was my first play date apart from my parents. Lunch went smoothly, but when the mother offered us milk, she said: "Do you want chocolate or white?" The words bumped up against my soul with a thud. I knew I was supposed to turn down the chocolate. I had specifically heard Mom say chocolate milk was not good for us. That's all I knew, but when my friend called out for chocolate, I did too.

I remember being surprised to see it was a far-from appealing brown color. Normally I would have turned up my nose at it, but the fact that this one thing was outlawed from my house made me think I should try it while I could. I drank it, just a sip at first, and then the whole glass and it tasted very good (of course) to my tongue, but the decision began to eat away at my soul. The voice of conscience echoed through my mind. I could not think, and barely noticed after lunch when they showed me their new color TV. When my mother showed up at the door to bring me home, guilt shivered through my whole being.

I did not know the term, but I recognized that I had sinned, and that I was now a sinner. I had never heard of salvation, but at the moment it seemed like there was none to be found. I had thrown off the innocence of childhood, tumbled into a state of uncertainty, lost the omnipresent sense of a loving God, and took my place among The Lost.

> If it had not been for the law, I would not have known sin. For I would not have known what it is to covet if the law had not said, "You shall not covet." But sin, seizing an opportunity through the commandment, produced in me all kinds of covetousness.
>
> For apart from the law, sin lies dead. I was once alive apart from the law, but when the commandment came, sin came alive and I died.
>
> *Romans 7:7 ESV*

You too, were once alive apart from the law; but when the commandment came, sin became alive and you died. It's not just the ten commandments which awaken sin, but all the laws we make for ourselves: "Keep the portion size small." "Never take thirds." "Restrict carbs." "Don't snack." Those are all laws along the lines of "Do not covet." And they all serve to arouse and awaken sin.

GOODBYE TO LAW

Remember what happened when the Israelites encountered hardship in the wilderness? They thought it might be better back in Egypt where they were slaves. *(Exodus 16, Numbers 11).* Sigh. What does God have to do to convince us that liberty is better than slavery?

We know He has set us free from the law, but how many of us think that maybe…just maybe…adding this one little law won't hurt a thing and might actually slim me down?

The trouble is, when we seek to be justified by the law, we have fallen from grace.

> **Christ is become of no effect unto you, whosoever of you are justified by the law; you are fallen from grace.** *Galatians 5:4 KJV*

Serious business. How many Christians are aware that Christ has become of no effect for them, because they are trying to achieve perfection on their own strength? How many times have we rendered Christ inoperative, useless in our lives, by trying it our way?

Oh, the tears we should weep for our numbness of mind and cold, self-centered hearts. By clinging to our own devices, we hold His Spirit at arm's length.

> Now the Lord is the Spirit, and where the Spirit of the Lord is, there is freedom.
>
> *II Corinthians 3:17 ESV*

What laws are governing our lives? Are they overriding the Holy Spirit's whisper? As we begin our day, are we listening to a litany of self-imposed duties (I must read my Bible, I must walk three blocks, I must only eat two bowls of cereal) or are we listening for the gentle nudge of the Holy Spirit?

> For freedom Christ has set us free; stand firm therefore, and do not submit again to a yoke of slavery.
>
> *Galatians 5:1 ESV*

Yay, freedom!

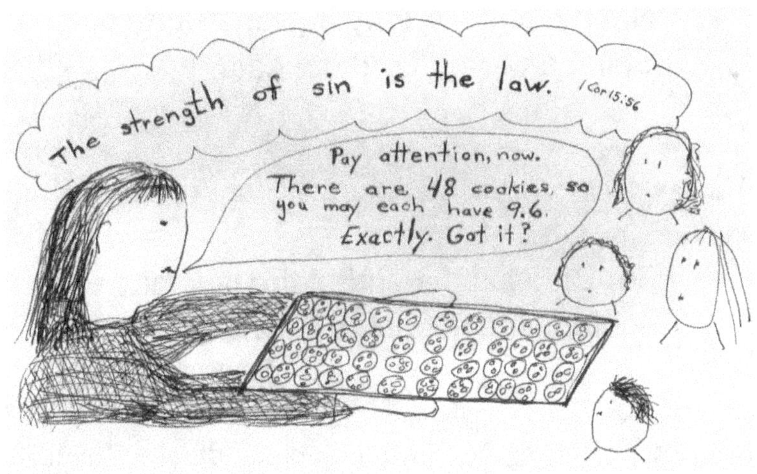

THE END OF THE LAW

Where there is no law there is no transgression.

Romans 4:15 ESV

As a child, up until some point, you knew how to eat. Then the laws—eat this, don't eat that, not so much, eat more of this, never before dinner—awakened sin to you, because:

The strength of sin is the law.

I Cori. 15:56 KJV

Yes, the law strengthens sin. Let that sink deep into your consciousness. Whatever it is that we try to avoid becomes the focus of our desire. Even if a person excels at willpower, eventually he will give in because he is relying upon the weak flesh, instead of the power of God.

Not by might, nor by power, but by my
Spirit, says the Lord of hosts.

Zachariah 4:6 ESV

The law awakens sin, yes. But that's not the end of the story, thank God.

For Christ is the end of the law for
righteousness to everyone who believes.

Romans 10:4 ESV

It's not by setting laws for ourselves that we achieve peace with food and with our bodies. It's by receiving His gift of righteousness, and walking in the Spirit.

By sending his own Son in the likeness of
sinful flesh and for sin, He condemned sin
in the flesh, in order that the righteous
requirement of the law might be fulfilled in
us, who walk not according to the flesh but
according to the Spirit.

Romans 8:2 ESV

The wonderful news is that we have the Spirit of God. We no longer strive in the flesh to accomplish the law. We simply trust and obey. How nice is that?

The law brings wrath, but where there is
no law, there is no transgression.

Romans 4:15 ESV

A GLIMPSE OF THE SPIRIT

> So I say, walk by the Spirit, and you will not gratify the desires of the flesh.   *Gal. 5:16 NIV*

For the first 20 years of my life, I was maybe the most un-Holy-Spirit-led person ever to exist on the Earth. No religious training whatsoever. I had no idea there was such a thing as a Holy Spirit.

That little nudge of God telling me, "Go here," or "Do that," I interpreted as temptation, something to overcome. Rather than allow God to guide my actions, I thought I was supposed to overpower these nudges, trusting solely in the power of mind.

I was continually grieving the Spirit of God, continually fighting with the peace that passes understanding. I had no idea who I was pushing away. I was one messed up kid.

AGE 12. I was old, yet hardly a teen, already weary of myself that day when the Spirit of God began to shake me awake.

I slogged along, wandering, my mind and emotions clogged with nothingness. It seemed apparent to me that I was abandoned and without hope; there was no way out for me. I was stuck being me. And me, I recognized, was inherently, irrevocably flawed.

The accusing thoughts began again; these voices that had criticized me for half my life: I was fat. I ate too much sugar. I was getting fatter. And they were right. They were all right.

At that moment the weight of all those years of self-criticism came crashing down on me, and I collapsed there in the field, crying out in my disgust at my own selfishness and lust, acknowledging the truth in those voices to whomever would hear (if perhaps there was someone up there who could hear). In that heart cry came the answer. I was immediately soothed by a comforting Presence, dissolving every fear.

Feeling a gentle pull to stand and follow, I went along attentively, not knowing where It was taking me, but trusting this thought that had instantaneously brought peace.

This Presence took me to an emerald-green moss-covered mound, a glorious place where the last of the sun still shone; a place I had never seen before though I knew the field well. I had no doubt that it was Love that brought me here, Someone who loved me more than I loved myself.

I had no name for this being, but when I obeyed His leading I had confidence, I knew what to do and where to go; and when I did not, I returned to the restless world of darkness. I had felt these gentle tugs times before, but I had disregarded them as not worthy of my attention.

With great shame I realized now I had been pushing away the Creator, trampling upon His Spirit even as it beckoned me to come.

> For all who are led by the Spirit of God
> are sons of God.   *Romans 8:14 ESV*

Having no root or support or even any words for what had happened, it didn't stick with me long. I let the Thought slip, went my own way within hours, and put aside the experience entirely. Fierce trials over the course of many years ensued before I would accept this gentle leading for my life as the only Way. Many horrifying situations followed before I could acknowledge, once and for all, my absolute need and before I would freely offer myself to God.

IT'S BEEN NAILED TO THE CROSS

It's a secret so profound, that to discover it is to feel like you've been born again again.

> Now in Christ Jesus you who once were far off have been brought near by the blood of Christ. For He Himself is our peace, who … has broken down in his flesh the dividing wall of hostility by abolishing the law of commandments expressed in ordinances.
>
> *Ephesians 2:13 ESV*

Do you understand those blessed words? Christ abolished the law of commandments and all its ordinances through His suffering and death. All its ordinances. The regulations made by God were abolished at the cross.

Clearly I remember the transforming moment years later when in my kitchen God spoke to me—that Christ was the end of every law, even the laws of my own making. Every the diet rule I struggled under was abolished. Every picky and not-so-picky rule I had set for myself were nailed to the cross. The rules about portion size and fattening foods and what to eat and when. Nailed to the cross. He spoke to my heart: They are no longer your master. You are free.

Settle that in your heart. Meditate on it. You are free. To be led by the Spirit is to be free.

CALLED TO FREEDOM

For you were called to freedom, brothers.
Galatians 5:13 ESV

Satan hates freedom, so he's telling you even now that some rules are good and you can't do without them. He may be whispering to you that, as an example, it's a good rule that you don't eat poison; which is of course true. But of course it is a silly argument, because neither will the Holy Spirit lead you to eat poison. Satan may be whispering that it's a good rule to not eat the whole gallon of ice cream, but neither will Christ lead you to eat that. You don't need rules.

Suppose I make a rule "no sweets." I think I can lose weight by not eating anything with refined sweets, so no more sweets. I inscribe the rule on my forehead. Then I am hungry at work one day, and there they are in the break room looking all appealing—dark chocolate brownies—and with nothing else to eat, I grab one. Tasting it, I feel condemned. I am afraid to even look to God. I feel like I am bad. And because I am feeling bad, I find myself eating another and later another, hiding the crumbs, wallowing in the darkness of self-doubt and despair. But really I was just hungry.

Had I not set the no-sweet rule for myself, I would have the peace of Christ. I would have been able to pass right by them without a second thought, or I would have eaten with thanksgiving and a clear conscience. It is not so important what you eat or don't eat. God is not obsessed with what you eat. He can work around it. What God doesn't like is idolatry, both the idolatry that says "I have to have this NOW" and the idolatry that says "I must be THIN no matter what." He doesn't like it when you worry, because worry is the enemy of health. That which does not spring from faith is sin.

> **Whoever has doubts is condemned if he eats, because the eating is not from faith. For whatever does not proceed from faith is sin.** *Romans 14:23 ESV*

Eat in faith, holy beloved of God, and thank Him for everything that crosses your palate. If as you look to Him you feel led to eat it, thank God for it. Ask Him to bless it and use those calories for His Kingdom. Everything created by God is good.

Remember the little kid song, "We are weak and He is strong." It's true. It is only when we admit we are confused and unreliable, unable to stand against the evil one alone, unable to save ourselves from the lusts of the flesh…it is only then that the power of God becomes available to us.

> **When I am weak, then I am strong.** *II Corinthians 12:8 ESV*

It is such a relief to share our weakness and our worries and our sorrows and our burdens with the One who fixes everything!

The Lord longs for us to trust Him:

> Trust in the Lord with all your heart, and do not lean on your own understanding. In all your ways acknowledge Him, and He will make straight your paths. Be not wise in your own eyes; Fear the Lord, and turn away from evil. It will be healing to your flesh and refreshment to your bones.
>
> *Proverbs 3:5 ESV*

Did you catch that? Healing to your flesh! Refreshment to your bones! Who wouldn't want that? So what do we need to do to get it?

Trust in the Lord with all our heart. God will precisely direct us even in the little things. Keeping our eyes and our hearts fixed on Christ, we will learn His ways. And His ways are so much higher than our ways.

> As ye have yielded your members servants to uncleanness and to iniquity unto iniquity; even so now yield your members servants to righteousness unto holiness.
>
> *Romans 6:19 KJV*

That's what it means to fear the Lord. That's what it means to be led by the Spirit. And that's where we'll find healing and refreshment for our bones. Hallelujah!

THE PURPOSE OF WILLPOWER

One might ask, "If willpower doesn't work, then why do we have it?" Good question.

Perhaps it is true that willpower is the one attribute of man that separates us from animals. If that is the case, it would explain why humans have made such a mess of the world, and animals have not. Humans, in following our own wills, have continually resisted the will of God.

Why then was mankind ever endowed with such a thing as a will? This much I know. God is Love. And He wants us to share His nature. Thus:

> **God has shut up all in disobedience so that He may show mercy to all.**
>
> *Romans 11:32 NAS*

Our Loving Heavenly Father wants us to experience His mercy so that we too can become the embodiment of mercy as He is. In order to experience His mercy, we had to need His mercy. And for that, we had to have a will.

So what is the purpose of the will now that we are saved? The will's job is to grab all those runaway thoughts that occur to us and bring them into subjection to Christ. The will's purpose is to take hold of every wayward desire and present it to a Living God. The will's purpose is to turn our errant heart over again and again to the transforming power of the Living Word, Jesus Christ.

Thank you Holy God.

THEY CALLED HIM A GLUTTON

If you think you're alone, you're not. Jesus knows what you're suffering. He's been there. In every way you are tempted, He was tempted.

> For we do not have a high priest who is unable to sympathize with our weaknesses, but one who in every respect has been tempted as we are, yet without sin.
>
> *Hebrews 4:15 ESV*

And people called Him a glutton.

> John came neither eating nor drinking, and they say, "He has a demon." The Son of Man came eating and drinking, and they say, "Look at Him! A glutton and a drunkard."
>
> *Matthew 11:18 ESV*

The Pharisees criticized John for fasting so much; and they criticized Jesus for eating so much. We always see skinny pictures of Jesus, but it's possible maybe He wasn't always so skinny. Jesus was at one point called a glutton.

Being called a glutton is not fun for anybody. Maybe you've never been called a glutton in so many words, but the way people look at you, their judgment of your eating habits, their rejection of who you are, has left you tattered and beaten and scarred But not for life.

Behold, I am making all things new.

Revelation 21:5 ESV

We actually don't know why they called Jesus a glutton, but we do know this: He was not a glutton. He was utterly sinless, yet He was ridiculed for his eating. He faced rejection and sensitivity to what people were thinking…all the same temptations we face. He was overwhelmed with the desire to drown his sorrows in overeating, but He did not—never ever—sin.

Because Jesus experienced temptation when He suffered, He is able to help others when they are tempted. *Hebrews 2:17 GNT*

Our God knows. He has been there. He faced what you face, He endured the temptations you and I endure. He suffered more than any man, the Bible says, and faced the ultimate rejection.

HOW DID I GET THIS WAY?

I became a glutton to numb my senses. The effect was always temporary, and as soon as I came to my senses there was never any doubt I had just added to my struggles, and not solved anything. This was me:

> For although they knew God, they neither glorified Him as God nor gave thanks to Him, but they became futile in their thinking and darkened in their foolish hearts.... Therefore God gave them up in the lusts of their hearts to impurity, to the dishonoring of their bodies…to dishonorable passions.
>
> *Romans 1:19 NAS*

I'm sure this Scripture describes exactly what happened to me. Every time I turned away from God, He allowed me to wallow in my own lusts, and I spiraled downward from one awful sin to another headlong to my own destruction. Meanwhile, He reached for me.

> "All the day long I have stretched out my hands to a disobedient and obstinate people."
>
> *Romans 10:21 ESV*

How many times did God reach to hug me and I turned away? Those years of painful torment, the overpowering lusts that ate away at everything good in my life, through it all I was simply reaping the fruit of my own way.

Daddy God, help us to listen! Help us to want to listen!

ALONE

Let's be real. When you love food so much that it gets in the way of living, it's become your god. And that's the way it was for me for more years than I care to remember:

AGE 16. The aloneness jumped out at me, gnawed at my insides the moment I stepped in the door.

Our two-story white farmhouse was tucked away in a remote valley in upstate New York. Houses were few and far between. Dad was gone on business again, for weeks, months: his return too far distant to anticipate. The only neighbors were coarse-talking— kids who called people "niggers" and threw stones at birds.

My older sister—the one person who could bolster my courage—had flown off to college in Ohio; and now, as a final stab to my soul, my mother had accepted a job miles away in Syracuse. No longer would I find her awaiting my return from school, ironing at the ironing board, attentive to my stories of the day. She was a stockbroker now, in wool suits trying to find acceptance in a man's world. My whole life consisted of Mom and me, and Mom wouldn't be home until long after the dull gray hours of afternoon had worn away to evening. The farmhouse creaked.

The only way I knew to turn off the loneliness was to eat....

So it came to be that once off the bus and inside the front door, food was everything and all that I sought. For hours, I searched one cupboard to the next, from the top of the refrigerator to the bottom of the freezer, grazing off everything sweet or crispy or starchy or salty that I found, and when I finished the rounds of the kitchen, I would start all over again.

I shaved off a little here and scooped out the edges there, masquerading the parts I had removed by fluffing up the part that was left. When I emptied a container, I plunged it deep into the garbage to hide it from sight. When the can began to overflow, I dumped its contents on the floor and reorganized the trash, placing the empty packages I had consumed on the bottom, in hopes that my mother would forget they had ever existed. Sometimes, it worked.

But there were days—and this was one of those days—where even camouflaging my eating seemed like too much work. Gorging, devouring, inhaling, I ate cookies and pound cake and jelly bread and ice cream bars and frozen cookie dough and everything and anything I could find that was sweet or salty. I consumed the entire container of marshmallow ice cream and stuffed potato chips in my mouth until I couldn't stand them anymore.

Then I guardedly took out the butter pecan ice cream, a flavor I despised, and ate it anyway because it was sweet and creamy and I hoped it would stop up the emotions that were screaming within me.

When the ice cream had melted to stickiness and was mostly gone, I returned to the three-gallon potato chip can and began stuffing one after another into my mouth scratching my throat with the hardly chewed pieces. I had developed a system—eat as much salty food as I could devour until I grew sick of it, then as much sugary food as I could stand until it revolted me, then go back to salty foods until I could eat no more, sugary, salty, swapping back and forth in a desperate attempt to fill the aching void.

I was horribly overstuffed, but I continued gorging. I wanted with every part of my being to stop, but I kept on. I ate everything in sight until my swollen and distended stomach churned in rebellion, the food started backing up my throat, and I got a glimpse of the hell I was creating for myself.

At that moment the selfish slob I was became clear: fingers stuck together with ice cream goo, potato chip and cake crumbs poking at my neck and drizzled under my blouse, the kitchen now bare and robbed of groceries, and every cell in my body bloated with gluttony.

As the digestive contents fought to be heaved out, a holy enlightenment fell on me, revealing the disgusting broken mess of my heart. I fled to the kitchen window, looked over the green meadows which told of the peace I had ignored, and there I cried out from the depths of my soul to the Creator, the Almighty, the Whoever, to save me, rescue me from this self-destruction. From a place of utter humiliation, from the deepest chasm of my heart, I called out, "Please help me! Oh Whoever You Are, help me to get free, and someday I'll help other people to get free."

And then there was calm.

I cleaned up the kitchen. Mom never said a word.

A LESSON

It was a banana-eating contest—the high school youth group pitted against their Sunday school teacher. The bleachers in the gym were full of interested onlookers, family and friends. I never learned who had issued the challenge, but whoever could eat the most bananas in three minutes would win, the. five students averaging their consumption.

Both groups looked healthy. Both looked eager and excited to get started: the teacher perhaps slightly less so. The two teams were separated by a screen so neither could see the other, but from the bleachers we could watch both sides.

A bell rang to start the contest and, even though I had known what to expect, I couldn't believe my eyes. Instantly the teacher began peeling and downing bananas one after another, peeling and downing, obviously enjoying the crowd's approval, and gleeful at the thought of beating the youth group. As his pile of peels grew, he continued devouring huge bites and peeling the next one.

The crowd's laughter began to strike me as a bit strange, and I looked over at the students. Wait a minute, they weren't stuffing bananas in their mouths. Hidden from the teacher's view, they were calmly sitting and smiling, each holding a banana. Sometimes one or the other would take a bite from the banana, enjoying the taste, and slowly pull the peel down a bit farther. Not one of the kids had finished even one banana.

Three minutes passed, the buzzer sounded, the teacher threw up his hands and the master of ceremonies counted the peels he had left on the floor.

The Sunday School teacher had eaten 15 whole bananas. The audience was going wild, clapping profusely, and rose to give a standing ovation, but it wasn't until the screen was drawn back that the teacher understood who they were clapping for. We were clapping for the courageous students, who had known better than to eat more than their bodies could use.

> Do you not know that your body is a temple of the Holy Spirit within you, whom you have from God? You are not your own, for you were bought with a price. So glorify God in your body. *I Corinthians 6:19 ESV*

CHAPTER 3
THE GIFT OF REPENTANCE

Their end is destruction, their god is their belly, and they glory in their shame, with minds set on earthly things. *Phil. 3:19 ESV*

Thank God thank God for the gift of repentance. What a joy to repent and be cleansed! Sometimes I'm stubborn, seeking after pleasures instead of purity, looking for satisfaction in stuff instead of Spirit. Then I remember something in the Word of God, and …oh.

There are times I persist in justifying myself instead of just repenting, my heart filled with pride. Like the children of Israel, I've demanded my own way, my own choice of food, relying on my own understanding…and His Word brought me up short each time. Over the years, I've been hit up the side of the head with this Scripture a good many times:

Do not be deceived: God is not mocked, for whatever one sows, that will he also reap.
Galatians 6:7 ESV

The Word of God wounds that it may heal. A stream of water can carve a jagged rock smooth and break up boulders into soil, so the Word of God can transform even the stone-cold heart into fertile ground for His Spirit. How good it is to let the His Word flood our minds and hearts! What joy can match the cleansing joy of true repentance?

POWER IN WEAKNESS

> My power is made perfect in weakness.
> Therefore, I will boast all the more gladly
> of my weaknesses, so that the power of
> Christ may rest upon me.   *II Cor. 12:9 ESV*

AGE 17 I was one who hated to be seen eating, wondering what people thought of me. "Do they think I'm eating too much?" "Am I eating too much?" "Will they think I'm greedy?" However, at age 17 I finally took the first step toward honesty. I admitted my weakness for everyone in the family to see.

I set up a chart on the wall to keep track of my weight, and labelled it boldly "Mary's Fat Leg Chart". Putting the numbers there in plain sight was a brave move in a household where, frankly, no one admitted ever having a problem with anything. It was a start in the right direction.

But I soon found focusing on the number of pounds I weighed was not going to stop me from eating too much, nor bring me peace.

Nevertheless, something wonderful did happen as a result. My parents decided to put our whole family on a diet they read about in the newspaper. I remember we ate no bread, no potatoes, no starch, and no refined sugar. It was austere. I missed the bread, I missed the potatoes, but truthfully I did not miss the sugar. And within days I began to see the power of diet change. My mind was clearer. I woke up with energy.   I was smarter in school. The cravings, surprisingly, diminished or disappeared.

The family all lost ten or twenty pounds before my parents declared the diet over. I surprised myself by asking Mom not to go back to buying cookies and sweets as she had so regularly in the past. She objected at first, but my sincere plea touched her and she agreed.

I had learned the amazing truth that what you eat affects your mood and everything about you. It was a start.

Yes, we will confess our weaknesses, and we will be glad to do so! For in that confession is the sure acknowledgement of healing begun.

FOOD IS FOR THE STOMACH

Every Scripture has value. But occasionally, one will resound through your being and make your inner hairs stand up on end. That's the way it was for me with this Scripture.

> All things are lawful for me, but not all things are helpful. All things are lawful for me, but I will not be dominated by anything. Food is meant for the stomach and the stomach for food—and God will destroy both one and the other. I Corinthians 6:14 ESV

Food is for the stomach? Oh. It's such a simple concept, but one that had escaped me most of my life. I had never asked my stomach what it wanted to eat. I had always asked my mind. And my mind's idea of what to eat had little to do with the actual physical needs of my body.

Food is for the stomach? It's not for the mind, to soothe the hurts and turmoil of living? It's not for the tongue, to titillate the taste buds and set the saliva streaming? It's not for the eyes, just because it looks so yummy; or for the nose, because it has a fragrance that tantalizes? It's not for the teeth, for the crunchy goodness that biting down and chewing offers? FOOD IS FOR THE STOMACH!!! It was a revelation that absolutely and forever changed the way I thought about food.

Since that day I have learned not to ask my mind, "What do you want to eat?" I don't ask my taste buds, "What do you want to eat?" I go straight to my stomach, check in with it, and yes, the stomach knows best. The Holy Spirit restores that connection that was lost through sin and unbelief, and what a wonderful blessing that restored communication with your stomach is. Your amazing body will give you an indication of what it needs, and the Holy Spirit will help you determine what to eat.

If you're in the habit of feeding your taste buds, rather than your stomach, you are fighting a losing battle. There are thousands of taste buds in your mouth, and not one of them will ever say, "Enough." The stomach, on the other hand, has much more reasonable demands, requesting only food to sustain health and keep you active. With this realization, my desires began to shift. I began to like the foods that before I had barely tolerated. I began to understand what food was for.

Food is for the stomach. As long as the stomach is content, don't let your eyes tell you, "OOO! That looks good!" … or your mind cry out, "Oh! I just have to try that!" …. or your emotions say, "I deserve a little treat now and then." Don't let your taste buds rule your life. "Oh! But I know it's going to taste so good!" Submit the desire—this desire and every desire—to the Lord. And let the Holy Spirit lead. Maybe He will lead you to eat it; maybe not. But you know He'll lead you to something which will actually satisfy. Our gracious Creator knows exactly what will hit the spot.

LUNCHTIME AT CENTRAL SCHOOL

AGE 15-18. It was lunchtime at Central. The noise of hundreds of highschoolers boomed with intensity, echoing off the walls of the lunchroom. The din of voices sharply offended my need for quiet so at lunchtime, while the rest of the school talked and laughed, I chose to eat alone as far away from the noise as possible.

My breakfast had been scanty: one little bowl of puffed rice and as much sugar as I could add without visibly emptying the sugar bowl. Ravenous by lunch time, I picked at the instant mashed potatoes, inhaled the milk, gobbled the perennial apple crisp, then covered the unappealing meat and canned vegetables with a napkin and returned the tray.

I hated returning the tray because it set me front and center, back turned, in view of the whole school. Each day as I walked to deposit my tray, I tried what I could to prevent the world from noticing my expanded rear end.

That was my lunch day after day, week after week, until one day I noticed a table of some of the quieter people I knew. I sat down across from Francine—who was enviably lean and healthy—and watched her open her lunchbox and take out a whole tuna sandwich, a half peanut butter sandwich, carrots, and an apple. Some days she bought an ice cream bar too. How could she eat so much and be thin?

Then I focused my attention on a couple of healthy-looking boys whom I admired, not because of their good looks, but because they got up from the table looking satisfied. For several days in a row I gazed on these two boys right at the moment they finished eating, grabbed their spent lunchboxes, and rose from the table. Never did I detect even a hint of craving on their faces. To be like them! Those boys gave the impression they were absolutely and completely satisfied. Not stuffed. Just satisfied. No lingering longings. They ate, and when they were done eating, they got up satisfied and went off to toss a football or whatever they went off to do.

This was I think my junior year in high school, and to my knowledge I had never risen from that table or any table with a feeling of being satisfied. There were plenty of times at home I had eaten to the point of being over-stuffed—in which case I marinated in the bitter juices of remorse for several hours afterward. More often I stood up with a lingering longing for carbohydrates, wanting, desiring, plotting how I might sneak more throughout the evening without being observed. But never did I remember being satisfied.

That these boys, or anyone in the world, could eat and feel satisfied was a revelation, and awakened in me a longing for this glorious contentment. That day I resolved to search until I found the key to a peaceful relationship with food.

My quest for satisfaction took me through torturous episodes of gluttony, years of white-knuckle deprivation, and into the horrors of Satan's pharmacy. Then, floundering in the nothingness of Eastern religion, my body slithered into anorexia, a condition that left me helpless, weak, and still no closer to freedom.

If God had not intervened.... Anorexia may sound good to some of you who idolize the idea of being thin. But anorexia is only this—the fear of eating—and your internal organs, faced with shortages, shut down one by one. Mine were seizing up before the day finally came when I found the peace beyond understanding. I finally came to the end of my self-led, futile and frightful journey, and began a new one holding the hand of God. It was there that I learned how to eat.

THE ULTIMATE COUNSELOR

"From any tree of the garden you may eat freely; but from the tree of the knowledge of good and evil you shall not eat, for in the day that you eat from it you will surely die."
Genesis 2:17 NAS

Laws by nature are designed to fail, even when enacted by ourselves on ourselves. Even as Adam and Eve chose to disobey the one rule—one little rule—they had been given, we find ourselves transgressing every little law we set for ourselves. "I'll only eat at mealtimes." "I'll keep portion sizes small." "I'll never take seconds or thirds." "I'll only eat half this chocolate bar." The law, like the one little law given to Eve, triggers an anxious longing for what we cannot have. As a result, we fail, and discouragement is one of Satan's best tricks.

The fact is, sometimes we do need to eat thirds, and maybe fourths or fifths (or sixths!) of something. So why devise rules for ourselves that we can't, and don't need to, keep?

Think about it: How can you find that exact tuning of nutrients that you will actually feel like eating, that will fill you up completely, and that will at the same time reward your body with true health and fitness? Even if you counted every calorie and weighed out fat grams and moisture content, could you arrive at that precise arrangement of nutrients appropriate to your particular body type and energy output and environment?

The reality is uncomfortable to accept, but the fact is you and I have so little knowledge of the precise blend of nutrients our bodies need in order to be totally satisfied and completely healthy at any point in time that we will never be able to get it exactly right.   There is always going to be a tension between what we are telling our bodies to eat and what our bodies want to eat.   Or is there?

> **But Jesus looked at them and said, "With man this is impossible, but with God all things are possible."** *Matthew 19:26 ESV*

What man can't do, God can. We will never be able to figure out exactly what foods in what quantities eaten at what time would be best for us, but the Great Shepherd of our souls knows exactly what we need, and He is more than willing to lead us to eat just that. The Lord God will take over where we leave off. In so far as we are willing to abandon our own will, the Lord and Savior Jesus Christ will come and fill us. He alone can satisfy us and at the same time bring us into the best of health.

Why do so many Christians of all shapes and sizes still live with continual doubt and frustration about their eating, craving what they think they shouldn't eat, failing in the attempt to stop bingeing, and beating themselves up for the fact that they are overweight? Our loving

Savior is absolutely understanding. Paul expresses the frustration of one who is under the law:

> For I know that nothing good dwells in me, that is, in my flesh. For I have the desire to do what is right, but not the ability to carry it out. For I do not do the good I want, but the evil I do not want is what I keep on doing.
>
> *Romans 7:15 ESV*

Every one of us has been there, but we don't have to stay there! That's the point. Our friend Paul continues:

> O Wretched man that I am! Who will deliver me from this body of death? Thanks be to God through Jesus Christ our Lord!
>
> *Romans 7:24 ESV*

Who will deliver? Christ will! Christ in us, the hope of glory! Help freely given. Our Loving Father doesn't want us to be overweight. Yahweh does not want us to be anxious and guilty for overeating. It is to His Glory that we are healthy and full of life, satisfied all day long. God delights to satisfy us! God delights in making us young-looking, fit and active. He delights in our wholeness and victory over temptation! And He has provided the answer through the death and resurrection of His Son and infilling of the Holy Spirit.

> You will receive power when the Holy Spirit comes on you.
>
> *Acts 1:8 NIV*

TO WAIT UPON THE LORD

What would happen if you and I refused to move until we felt the leading of God?

> **The Lord is good to those who wait for Him, to the soul who seeks Him.** *Lam. 3:25 ESV*

This is God's will for you and for me. This is the Spirit-controlled life. Instead of jumping in and rushing off to do our own will, we humble ourselves and wait for Him to initiate.

> **Wait for the Lord; be strong, and let your heart take courage; wait for the Lord!**
> *Psalms 27:13 ESV*

We wait for him before speaking. We wait for him before eating. We wait for him as we shop. "But it seems so time consuming," you think. "I don't have time to wait on the Lord." You don't have time NOT to wait upon the Lord.

> **Wait for the Lord and keep his way, and He will exalt you.** *Psalms 37:34 ESV*

If you want a good outcome, if you don't want to waste your time on this Earth, wait on Him. The outcome is guaranteed when you let Christ be the One driving force in your life, not just in a general sense, but in every little detail. We must be faithful in the little decisions if we would like Him to help us with the big ones.

It is impossible to be led by God in the big things if you are not willing to be led by God in the small.

You see, it matters how you wear your hair. It matters what clothes you put on. It matters how you treat your dog. And it matters what you buy at the grocery store. It matters where you sit in church. It all matters.

And it takes courage to wait on the Lord. You have to be willing to look foolish. You have to be willing to do whatever the Spirit wills, outcome unknown. You have to be willing to trust the One who rules the universe and all things, the One who knows exactly the best way.

So sweet is the salvation of Our God.

CHAPTER 4
THE SECRET TO LIFE

> Walk by the Spirit, and you will not gratify
> the desires of the flesh.   *Gal. 5:16 ESV*

All right, okay. I need to walk by the Spirit. But how?

The first and most powerful thing you can do is to recognize you are dead.

That's right. Dead. When Christ died for sin, you died.

Why is that important? Because dead people don't sin. Sin no longer has power over you because you died.

> We know that Christ, being raised from the
> dead, will never die again; death no longer
> has dominion over him. For the death He
> died He died to sin, once for all, but the life
> He lives He lives to God. So you also must
> consider yourselves dead to sin and alive
> to God in Christ Jesus.   *Romans 6:9 ESV*

We are dead. Yahoo! Dead to all the temptations Satan can throw at us. Dead to all the guilt he could ever throw our way. You are dead. Christ is alive in you! Hold on to those words like treasure. I am dead to sin, but alive to God! Yes! Yes! Bless you Lord Jesus!

THANK GOD I'M DEAD

Greedy. I was greedy. I coveted even when I didn't want to. I wanted things I didn't even want. I couldn't share without wanting it back. Greed was rooted deep inside me. Every effort of the will could not loose its hold.

Until I realized I was dead.

> Do not be deceived: neither the sexually immoral… nor the greedy, … will inherit the kingdom of God.
>
> And such were some of you. But you were washed, you were sanctified, you were justified in the name of the Lord Jesus Christ and by the Spirit of our God.
>
> *1 Cor. 6:9 ESV*

That's the last word on greed. It's dead. You are alive.

When you gave your life to Christ, you died. There will be no more death. Someday you will leave your body behind, but not to worry—you've already died.

> We know that our old self was crucified with Him.
>
> *Romans 6:6 ESV*

It's a fact. When Christ was mocked, whipped, beaten, spat upon, tortured and crucified, we were in Him.

> For you have died, and your life is hidden with Christ in God.
>
> *Colossians 3:2 ESV*

We have died. What glorious and wonderful news! The power of sin has been dealt a death blow within us. You and I are free. We have died to the law. It is done.

> **Likewise, my brothers, you also have died to the law through the body of Christ....**
> *Romans 7:4 ESV*

Settle that within yourself. We have not just died to the Ten Commandments, but we've died to every law, every do-good principle that could flit upon our consciousness. Not only have we died to the multitude of laws of the Old Testament, including "Thou shalt not covet," but we have also died to every law we thought ourselves accountable to. We have died to "Thou shalt not take seconds (or thirds or fourths)," and we have died to "Thou shalt rise from the table when thou art still hungry." We have died to, "Thou must not ..." in all its forms.

Laws rely upon the pitifully weak self-will for their accomplishment, rather than on the amazing power granted us by the Spirit of God. Cravings aren't going to go away by thinking, "Thou shalt not covet. I will not covet. I must not covet," in all its forms. They go away when we reckon ourselves dead to sin.

His power is granted us to do <u>His</u> will at His timing in His way. If, seeking to live under dietary laws, we do by willpower manage to control our eating for a little while, what happens? A little pride creeps in. And then...whoops. Now we're right back where we started—feeling guilty again. Neither pride nor guilt is God's desire for us. He through His Son provided a better way.

> **He forgave us all our trespasses, having canceled the debt ascribed to us in the decrees that stood against us. He took it away, nailing it to the cross!** *Col. 2:14 NAS*

Perhaps you are thinking it can't be true. That was my response when I first began to understand what the Bible says about law, and the infinitely superior replacement, grace. The idea of abandoning the ceaseless struggle to obey God's laws seemed too good to be true. What about all the other laws I tried to live by, like: "read the whole Bible in one year," "pray an hour a day," "fast one day a month"? How could I live without those laws? What would prevent me from going into sin or falling astray?

Well, as I thought about it, I realized I wasn't doing too well with those laws. Especially the fasting. I was starting to resent God for making me work so hard to be a Christian. Something was wrong with my thinking. Gradually my mind began to receive what Paul had to say in the book of Romans:

> **Likewise, my brothers, you also have died to the law through the body of Christ, so that you may belong to another, to Him who has been raised from the dead, in order that we may bear fruit for God.** *Rom. 7:4 ESV*

Died to the law?

> While we were living in the flesh, our sinful passions, aroused by the law, were at work in our members to bear fruit for death. But now we are released from the law, having died to that which held us captive, so that we serve in the new way of the Spirit and not in the old way of the written code.
>
> *Romans 7:5 ESV*

Yes, the Law used to hold me captive. Like a stranglehold. And now God says I am released from the Law because I died? That Christ lives in me! God is saying that it's not up to me any more? Can this be?!!!

> Sin is no longer your master, for you no longer live under the requirements of the law. Instead, you live under the freedom of God's grace. *Romans 6:12 ESV*

The freedom of God's grace. Over and over again throughout the Bible, God is saying "Let Me." Scripture after Scripture points out the delusion of trying your best—which is never good enough. Instead, God yearns for us to admit our helplessness and fall entirely to rest in His arms. On our own we can do nothing.

> I am the vine; you are the branches. Whoever abides in Me and I in him, he it is that bears much fruit, for apart from me you can do nothing. *John 15:5 ESV*

Breathe that in: Apart from Jesus you can do nothing. It's fresh air to the soul. Our human nature is busy at work thinking of ways to lose weight—ways which have only a modicum of wisdom and may do more harm than good—and all the while God is so willing to lead and counsel, if we will only give the struggle up to Him.

All our striving just gets in the way of His perfect guidance. If God is leading me to eat the lunch I packed, but I think I should never eat lunch before eleven a.m., I am frustrating the Holy Spirit of God. If you obey the Lord's leading to eat that third bowl of granola now, you will find you're not stuck in the starved mode later, having to buy junk out of the machine just to get by.

Let God lead, brothers and sisters. Look to Him and let God lead. Dietary laws like "Thou shalt not eat..." actually awaken sin in us. Sin is inevitable when we live under the law. Let's read Romans 7:4 again:

> For while we were living in the flesh, our sinful passions, aroused by the law, were at work in our members to bear fruit for death. But now we are released from the law, having died to that which held us captive, so that we serve in the new way of the Spirit and not in the old way of the written code.
>
> *Romans 7:4 ESV*

Did you catch that? "Our sinful passions, aroused by the law." And that's not all!

The strength of sin is the law. *I Cor. 15:56 KJV*

What is the purpose of the Ten Commandments then? The Law of God served to show us our sin, so we would come to the Savior:

> **I would not have known what it is to covet if the law had not said, "You shall not covet."** *Romans 7:7 ESV*

Now, brought to the realization of our sin, we throw ourselves on the mercy of God, and through His Holy Spirit we find guidance and help in time of need.

> **For Christ is the end of the law for righteousness to everyone who believes.** *Romans 10:4 ESV*

Christ is the fulfillment of the law. He fulfilled every requirement on our behalf. The open, honest, and complete freedom that a little child feels—that is what Christ died to restore to us. Instead of trying and trying, we can simply trust.

> **Truly, I say to you, unless you turn and become like children, you will never enter the kingdom of heaven.** *Matthew 18:3 ESV*

How wonderful that we who have been born again through Christ can live as free as a child, tuned in to our Heavenly Father, always trusting in His unfailing love. Oh, the depth of the riches that are ours when we fall helpless upon the living God!

LUST IS LUST

It took me awhile to learn it, but now I know. Lust is lust. Lusty music, lusty clothing, lusty novels, lust for food…they're all tied together. Lust is lust.

Allowing our fantasies to run amok, allowing ourselves to covet just one thing, even a tiny thing, releases a power so significant it caused mankind's expulsion from the Garden of Eden.

That is the power of lust. Lust begins when the heart chooses its own way over God's way. And lust defiles.

> **"From within, out of the heart of man, come evil thoughts…and they defile a person."**
> *Mark 7:20 ESV*

The devil's desire is to steal the love which you have through the Holy Spirit, to kill the hope and confidence you have in Jesus Christ, and to destroy the childlike faith you have in the Heavenly Father.

This thief comes to make your life dull and mundane and demoralizing, even while he promises thrills and his slimy fulfillment. Christ came that we might have life!

> **The thief comes only to steal and kill and destroy. I came that they may have life and have it abundantly.**
> *John 10:10 ESV*

The Bible tells us what to do with lust. Flee!

> **Flee youthful lusts: but follow righteous-
> ness, faith, charity, peace.**   *2 Tim. 2:22 KJV*

Whenever we follow our heart and ignore the leading of God we end up in trouble. That's why God is continually calling us back.

> **Do not worship any other god, for the
> LORD, whose name is Jealous, is a
> jealous God.**   *Exodus 34:14 NIV*

The Lord God is jealous for you. Think of that. The King of kings and Lord of lords is jealous for you to return His love. Who else is so desirous of your affection?

God knows that He is the only one who can supply your need. He knows that He alone can soothe your suffering. The Lord Jesus Christ Himself longs for you with a godly jealousy:

> **I was crushed by their unfaithful heart
> which turned from me and by their eyes
> which lusted after their idols.** *Ezekiel 6:9 NET*

To Jesus, you are someone to die for.

GRACE

Actually there are two laws we are required to obey. #1:

> So speak and so act as those who are to
> be judged under the law of liberty.
> *James 2:12 ESV*

The law of liberty. Awesome, eh? But can you stand up to that judgment? Can you truly say you are walking in liberty? Or have you given yourself laws to obey, laws which restrict your freedom in Christ and bind you to the old sin nature?

And #2? Within the law of liberty is that special and wonderful law, which controls us:

> For the whole law is fulfilled in one word:
> "You shall love your neighbor as yourself."
> *Galatians 5:13 ESV*

I don't know about you, but I don't know how to do that without help from the Spirit of God. Likewise, we are to love the Lord our God with all our heart, all our soul, all our mind and all our strength. I don't know how to do that either. Thank God for the law of liberty. Thank God for His ultimate mercy. Thank God for the Spirit of God in us, recreating our hearts to love.

> God's love has been poured into our hearts
> through the Holy Spirit. *Romans 5:5 ESV*

THE DANCE

In the small high school I attended, I was president of the student council, editor of the school newspaper, and class salutatorian. My parents were a good example, and I can thank them for teaching me diligence, curiosity, independence, responsibility, and a million other things. But "be nice" was the extent of my religious training. The law of "be nice," of course, was hollow without Christ and would not save me from the horrors and the filth of giving away what should have been closely guarded for my future husband. By age 17 I was stained and broken. I began to earnestly seek God.

AGE 17. I can hear the hammering rock and roll music echoing from the school gymnasium as Mom drives off. The rock and roll of "Devil with the Blue Dress On" dominates the night air, and I have no real desire to go in.

But wait...a wisp of wind blows across my face and I catch the hint of a tiny melody in the distance. The raucous noise from the dance holds no attraction in comparison. I hope and wish for the delicate singing to persist long enough for me to trace it to the source, and I do—to the shabby wood-framed Pentecostal church across the way.

I step out of the chill winter winds into the drafty church and sit down in an empty pew. The 20 or so people there are singing with uplifted faces and raised arms, pouring their hearts out to a heavenly somebody I know nothing about. My hands grow cold, and then colder. It begins to dawn on me that the building has no heat. After a few more songs—and I am sitting on my hands to keep them warm—it can't be—but these poor souls are dipping people underwater! And everyone is cheering, so happy about the wet people, now wrapped in blankets.

They shout praises upward with gladness—the emotions are evidently real—and I leave with a feeling that I have glimpsed eternity.

Back at the dance I tell no one.

BURIED!

The word "baptize" in Greek is *baptizō,* and means to submerge, immerse, or dip under.

> Do you not know that all of us who have been baptized into Christ Jesus were baptized into his death? We were buried therefore with Him by baptism into death, in order that, just as Christ was raised from the dead by the glory of the Father, we too might walk in newness of life. *Romans 6:4 ESV*

Baptism is an outward sign of inward faith, but it is much more than that. Baptism is a recognition of the letting go of self. The old selfish self is finished; dead, gone forever.

> Baptism now saves you — not the removal of dirt from the flesh, but an appeal to God for a good conscience — through the resurrection of Jesus Christ. *I Peter 3:21 NAS*

Satan is still in the act of asking, "Has God said?" as he did in the Garden of Eden, and will surely try to tempt you to question whether you really are God's chosen child.

If you've been baptized since you believed, you can look back on that date and know that's the day you died. I don't care how much water you got up your nose, how silly you thought you looked sopping wet, and how insincere the preacher sounded—if you truly had a repentant heart before God, you were baptized with Christ. Satan cannot wash that memory from you. He may be able to wash other memories from you, but a sincere experience of baptism is one of those memories that sticks. Through Christ's death, you are dead to sin, buried with Him through baptism.

But that is not the end of the story!

> **I have been crucified with Christ. It is no longer I who live, but Christ who lives in me.** *Galatians 2:20 ESV*

You and I need never strive for acceptance with God again! The victory has been won. It is absolutely and completely finished! We need only abide in the love of God.

If you have been baptized into Christ, you can look back on that splashing of water, and know that you were made new. That simple act testifies that you were bought out of slavery, you were adopted, you belong to the I Am. Your spirit calls out Abba. You are one with Christ. You are loved. You are cherished. God Himself is your Dada. Nothing can separate you from His Love.

The story is written, and Christ has won. Our only job is to believe. And believe. And believe. And believe. And believe.

CHAPTER 5:
RIGHTEOUSNESS

> Put on the breastplate of righteousness.
> *Eph. 6:14 ESV*

"Righteousness?" you might say. "Not me. I'm not righteous. I could never be righteous."

And then maybe you think, "Well, I am praying more. Maybe I am a little righteous."

Don't go there. This breastplate of righteousness is not our righteousness. All our goodness adds up to one filthy disgusting heap in God's sight. The breastplate we are given is the breastplate of His righteousness. His righteousness we are freely given and His righteousness we are asked to wear.

His Righteousness. It is a privilege bestowed upon us when we believe. You are clean, you are justified, you are made right with God, thanks to His eternal sacrifice …one time…and for all. One of my favorite verses:

> You, who were dead in your trespasses and the uncircumcision of your flesh, God made alive together with Him, having forgiven us all our trespasses, by canceling the record of debt that stood against us with its legal demands. This He set aside, nailing it to the cross. *Colossians 2:14 ESV*

Nailing it to the cross. Can't you see it? The certificate of ordinances against us has been nailed to the cross. Eating more than we should? Nailed to the cross. Lying about it? Nailed to the cross. Stealing food? Nailed to the cross. Purging to eat more? Nailed to the cross. There is no more condemnation. You have been made acceptable in His eyes. You are beloved of God. It is done. You wear the breastplate of His Righteousness, knowing it was not earned. It is a gift of God's precious love poured out upon us at the cross. Wear that gift of His righteousness. It will guard your heart from the worst of what the enemy can throw your way.

SEATED WITH CHRIST

> God, being rich in mercy, because of the great love with which he loved us... raised us up with Him and seated us with Him in the heavenly places in Christ Jesus
>
> *Ephesians 2:4 ESV*

Yes, we are seated with Christ! It may not look like it to your earthly eyes, but we are! And the New Testament says that Jesus is seated far above all principalities and powers. *(Ephesians 1:21)* Far above! That's great news!

Of course, Satan doesn't want you to know it. He is trying hard to finagle his way into your thought life to get you to submit to a litany of rules: "do this", "don't do that." If he can get you to submit to those, he'll keep stepping up the demands, making it harder and harder for you to live with a clean conscience. Satan's goal, of course, is your discouragement. He wants you to give up on life and give up on Christ.

Does that make you mad? Yes, and it should!

> For the law of the Spirit of life in Christ Jesus has set you free from the law of sin and death.
>
> *Romans 8:2 ESV*

We are free in Christ Jesus. And we are seated with Christ far above every principality and authority and power and dominion, and above every name that is named in this age and the one to come. There's a beautiful view from up here.

UNDERSTANDING THE CONSCIENCE

You know how it went. Eve saw that the fruit was beautiful to look at. She saw that it was good to eat. And she believed Satan that it was desirable to make one wise.

Eve responded with the Word of God.   Or did she?

> The woman said to the serpent, "We may eat of the fruit of the trees in the garden, but God said, 'You shall not eat of the fruit of the tree that is in the midst of the garden, neither shall you touch it, lest you die.'"
>
> *Genesis 3:2 ESV*

Hold it. "Neither shall you touch it"? Where did that come from? That's not what God said.

> The LORD God commanded the man, saying, "You may surely eat of every tree of the garden, but of the tree of the knowledge of good and evil you shall not eat, for in the day that you eat of it you shall surely die."
>
> *Genesis 2:17 ESV*

So, was it Adam who added on the "no touch" rule? ("Look, Eve. Don't mess with that fruit. Don't even touch it.") Or did Eve concoct the no-touch rule on her own? In either case, the Scriptures point to the idea that someone added on to God's words.

"You won't really die," Satan said. And then maybe Eve touched it, and she didn't die. "Satan was right! I won't die!" But God had never said she couldn't touch it. He just said not to eat it.

Do you get the point? Don't add to the Word of God. Every confounded cotton-picking rule we have added on to God's Word, appealing as they seem, are of no value to improve our relationship with God. No value. None.

> These rules may seem wise because they require strong devotion, pious self-denial, and severe bodily discipline. But they provide no help in conquering a person's evil desires.
>
> *Colossians 2:23 NLT*

No help. Tattoo it on your brain. Inscribe it on your conscience. Stop adding on the Word of God. And step into the glorious freedom of Christ.

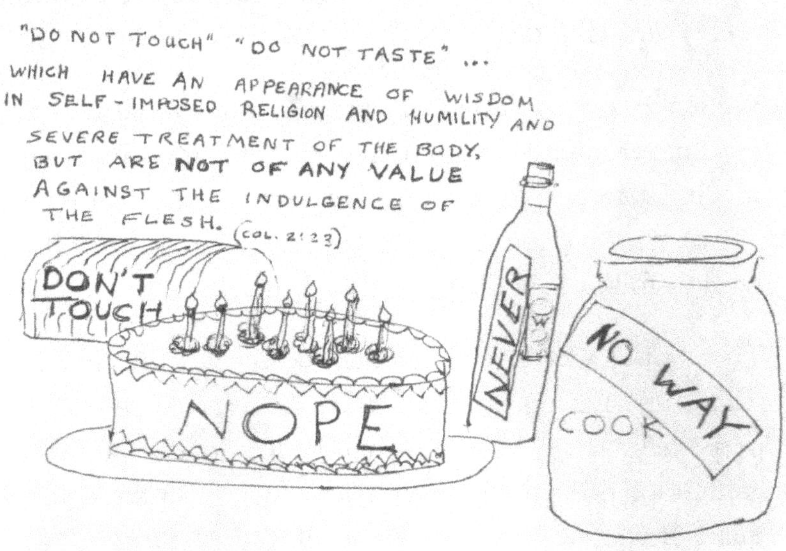

THE WHISPER IN YOUR EAR

I wonder. What would the world be like if Eve had understood from the beginning that it was okay to touch the fruit? In Eve's mind, once she touched it, she stood condemned. Satan would have been right there to whisper into her thought life, "You already sinned, so why not just go ahead and eat it?"

Likewise, Satan is right there to whisper the same taunt into your ear. "You know you shouldn't eat that handful of chips…you are a sinner for sure…you might as well go ahead and eat the whole bag….and then anything else you can find… there's no hope for you anyway." Like Eve, our consciences become defiled when we attempt to obey rules that are not of God.

> **To the pure, all things are pure, but to the defiled and unbelieving, nothing is pure; but both their minds and their consciences are defiled.** *Titus 1:15 ESV*

We make laws and rules for ourselves that God is not in, God never intended us to make, and that are sometimes much stricter than anything He would ask from us. Then, when we continually fall short, we think, "It is too hard to follow God. Why bother trying?"

Those of us who have been there know what it's like to wake up feeling stuffed and full and wretchedly perpetually fat. We know what it's like to assume there is no hope this side of heaven, so why not eat the whole quart of whipped topping for breakfast?

But hold on. Feeling bloated and full is not sin. It might just mean you should have eaten what you ate earlier in the day, so that your body would have time to digest before you went to bed.

Give this fat feeling to God, and look to Him for the answer. The Great Omnipotent God who lives within you can soothe that feeling of being overfull.

Look to Him. He might lead you to get some fresh air, eat some prunes, go for a walk. Remember, the fact that you feel full is not an indicator of sin. Sometimes it's just gas. When God convicts of sin, it is a heart issue. Your Heavenly Father is not looking at your bloated belly. He's looking at your heart.

A CLEAR CONSCIENCE

> Keep your faith and a clear conscience.
> Some men have not listened to their
> conscience, and have made a ruin of their
> faith.
>
> *I Timothy 1:19 NLT*

Conscience.   Such a blessed gift of God. But for years and years, my conscience was so demanding, so inflamed that no matter what I ate, I assumed a load of guilt afterwards.   I had a corrupted mind and a corrupted conscience.

> To the pure, all things are pure, but to those
> who are corrupted and do not believe,
> nothing is pure. In fact, both their minds
> and consciences are corrupted.
>
> *Titus 1:15 NIV*

The Holy Spirit's conviction is pure and right and wonderful. But when our conscience is full of rules we have set for ourselves, rules we read in a magazine, rules we heard from a friend, weight-loss tips we saw online, we are going to fail. We are unwittingly pitting ourselves against the Holy Spirit's leading.

As a child, I went through a period where I would kiss each of my stuffed animals good night. If I missed one or another, I would lie in bed worrying that they felt slighted. Similar is the condition of the Roman Catholic who feels compelled to pray to Mary. She might be exercising devotion, but the Spirit of God is not pleased with such sacrifices. *(I Timothy 2:5)* Without Christ, conscience is a heavy load.

God is always wanting to show us His lovingkindness through the wonderful blessings He provides, including the food we eat. But if we allow ourselves to feel guilty for everything we eat, how can He? Let us allow God to cleanse our consciences completely at the cross.

> **Since we have confidence to enter the holy places by the blood of Jesus…let us draw near with a true heart in full assurance of faith, with our hearts sprinkled clean from an evil conscience.** *Hebrews 10:19 ESV*

Ah, the glorious freedom we have in Christ! Our consciences become absolutely clean in the blood of Christ. We are no longer bound by rules that we cannot keep. Our only job is to walk step by step in the Holy Spirit, and this we can do by His grace. Hallelujah!

CONTENTMENT

Perhaps you are thinking: "Overeating doesn't really hurt anybody else except me, so I don't know why it's a big deal."

And that's a thought we've all had. But overindulging really is sin. Overindulging—not just in food, but in anything—is sin.

Why? Because God has created you for something better. Every moment spent outside the will of God is a moment when His Holy Spirit within us is grieved. Every moment spent chowing down in darkness is a moment God is not being formed in us, a moment we are not laying up treasures in heaven, a moment wasted.

> **Whoever knows the right thing to do and fails to do it, for him it is sin.** *James 4:17 ESV*

But how do we know what is the right thing to do? How do we know whether it's one cookie or eight cookies or fourteen thousand that we can eat? Or none at all?

One way: We look to Christ and trust the leading of His Spirit. It is hard sometimes, because you'll find God will lead you to eat a whole lot more of some things than you would ever guess—and at the same time lead you away from things you were accustomed to eating in the past—but over time you will learn to trust God's holy and peaceful leading confidently and without doubting.

Is the closet overflowing with clothes you thought would make you beautiful? Maybe the right shirt will cover my stomach. Maybe the right pants will make me look thin. But for the child of God, He gives more grace. Jesus lays it on the line:

> **Life is more than food, and the body more than clothing.** *Luke 12:23 NAS*

This is as practical as it gets. We think we need a new wardrobe to cover the unappealing aspects of our flesh, but He says Come to Me and I will make you beautiful.

If we'll allow the Lord entrance to the closets of our heart, He will undertake to do His work, reshaping us from the inside out. Your Heavenly Father knows precisely every need you have—from the zipper which is broken, to the pants that won't button, to the skirt that rides up—and as you deny yourself and really follow Him, everything (everything!) you need will, in perfect time, spring up before you and into your hands.

> **Godliness with contentment is great gain.** *I Timothy 6:6 ESV*

As we travel the course with Jesus at the helm, we begin to see the gradual transformation of our bodies into sanctified beautiful bodies, and our minds take on the beautiful contentment of Christ.

CHAPTER 6
HEADSTRONG

Not long after witnessing those church folk pouring out their souls in the cold to an invisible God, I felt called to surrender my life. And I did… almost. I knew I needed a Savior, there was no doubt, but I had no idea how capable the Savior really is.

AGE 17. High school graduation approaches and I am facing the fact that every scheme I have tried in my quest to be thin has been futile. I am considering getting into drugs, marijuana in particular, as a possible solution. But today, the rays of the sun dappling through the trees reach out to me. Mesmerized, I lift my heart in a desperate cry to the Creator of such beauty, Whoever that may be. It is a silent cry, but earnest, and I sense the Holy Presence. A gentle beckoning speaks to my heart, warmly inviting me.

Had I only accepted. The Door was open, salvation so close, and I almost did. But instead I imagine what it will be like trying to be a Christian, being around other Christians, and I am pretty sure that compulsive binge eating will eventually expose me as a sinner. Ordinary unbelief seems better than that. So I close my ears, turn away, and don't look back. I'll try marijuana instead.

I was sure that I needed to get control of this eating problem before I could come to Him. If I could just build up enough will power. Or if I just had the right technique, the right knowledge somehow, I could learn to eat.

I rejected God's offer, not knowing that Jesus came for people with incurable eating struggles like me. Jesus came for sin-sick folks like me.

> "Those who are well have no need of a physician, but those who are sick."
>
> *Matthew 9:10 ESV*

The ensuing years were a downward spiral, a journey dangling on the brink of extinction as I subjected my brain and body to alcohol, marijuana, LSD, hashish, and cocaine—all the while seeking freedom but only becoming more and more a servant of hell.

DEAD WORKS

It's one of the first principles in Christianity:

Repentance from dead works.

Therefore, leaving the principles of the doctrine of Christ, let us go on unto perfection; not laying again the foundation of repentance from dead works.

Hebrews 6:1 KJV

What are dead works? They are works we initiate. Works which seem good, but have no eternal value. Wood, hay, and stubble. They will all be burned.

Now if anyone builds on the foundation with gold, silver, precious stones, wood, hay, straw—each one's work will become manifest, for the Day will disclose it, because it will be revealed by fire, and the fire will test what sort of work each one has done.

I Corinthians 3:11 ESV

Is this you? You came to Christ years ago, but you're still trying to make yourself good. You try to eat less, maybe you fast, skipping meals to lose pounds, but you always fall back into overeating. That's what happens when you rely on self, on will power, on the flesh. Dead works.

Even though you know Jesus washed you from your sins, you feel like a sinner. It is an endless cycle: eat-guilt – don't eat – pride – overeat – guilt – on and on it goes. The cycle is designed by Satan to wear down the saints, and for a time, it has succeeded. *(Daniel 7:25)*

But let this revelation seep into your consciousness: the biggest problem you face is you—not the lustful-greedy you, but the rulemaking, tighten-up-the-ship, with-enough-effort-I-can-do-it you. The "good" you is the problem.

It's time to repent from the you that is working so hard to be good, to be right, to be thin. Why? Because when you trust that person to run the show, you are ignoring the One who actually knows how to make you good and right and thin. You have been acting on the opinion that God somehow doesn't know anything about eating. Dead works.

> **Go and learn what this means, 'I desire mercy, and not sacrifice.'** *Matthew 9:13 ESV*

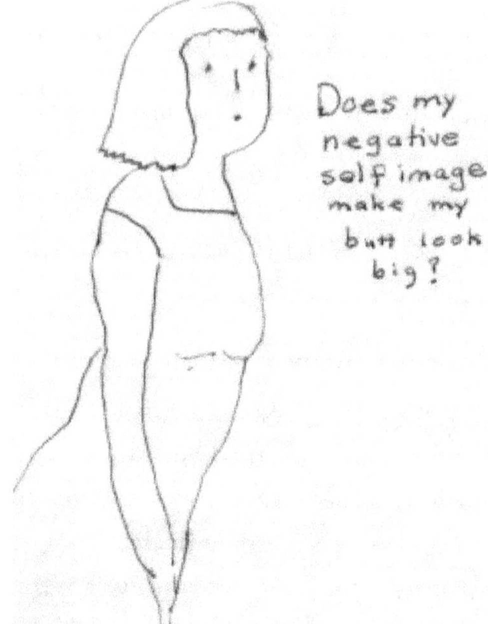

Man looks on the outward appearance,
but the Lord looks on the heart.

SUCKED IN: ANOREXIA

AGE 18-20: The blob that my body was becoming knew it was time to take action, so I started swimming at the college indoor pool. At first I could only swim diagonally across the corner of the pool, but the next time I could swim the whole way across the pool, and the next time I swam across and back. The wonderful feeling of floating invigorated me. Blood flow increased and improved my mental clarity. I became aware of my body in a new way. I began to be thankful for it, and instead of stuffing it with whatever tasted good, I began to appreciate it. I nourished it with food I thought would be good for it, plus whatever else I wanted to eat.

The dorm cafeteria system worked well for me, because for once I could eat as much as I wanted of everything and anything—cookies and ice cream and cake and pudding and wow. But—as is often the case—since there was no reason anymore to sneak, sweets lost some of their allure.

I realized I wasn't actually that fond of really gooey sweets, and found that I felt really good eating lots of salad and fish and even a vegetable here and there. I lost weight. But the reality is, I wouldn't have even tried the fish and the vegetables had I not been surrounded by people.

Because I was paranoid everyone anywhere near my table was scrutinizing my eating habits, analyzing my choices, and giggling under their breath whenever I ate too much, I did my best to show them I had no eating problem. Out of sheer embarrassment and shame, I almost never took seconds, ate only one dessert per meal, and spent minimal time in the cafeteria.

I did lose weight. I felt better and decided losing weight was the answer. So I cut back further and lost more weight. The pounds dropped off until my weight seemed just right. I was extremely happy! But the thought came to me that I better take off more, in case I should gain some back. Knowing my heart was still full of lust and greed, I thought it would be wise to lose as much as I could while I was still on a roll. So I continued to wrench myself from the table, in anguish leaving the cafeteria whenever the voice in my mind barked at me that I'd had enough.

And my mind would not relent. I was 128 pounds (58 kg), then 121 pounds (55 kg), and It kept dropping. I kept getting thinner and thinner. As long as my stomach was mostly empty, my conscience was quiet and I could feel good about myself, so I made sure it stayed empty.

You can't live that way. Eventually it will catch up with you. You'll either spiral back up the ladder or find yourself with debilitating health issues as I did. Near 100 pounds (45 kg), I began fainting from hunger in public places. I doubled over with pains in my heart. My body was breaking down.

So what does all this have to do with being led by the Spirit? Just this, I tried self-will. You could even say I won. I found I could ignore the internal cravings for food. Desire was conquered. But what good was it? I was dying. And I still didn't know how to eat.

LED BY THE FLESH
(KICKING AGAINST THE SPIRIT)

All these years I believed solely in the power of the will. Through sheer mental strength I thought I could overcome temptation. If I ever felt something like a spiritual leading, I fought against it.

That is the sickness of sin. I never imagined that the Holy Spirit could lead a person moment-by-moment. I had no idea I was fighting against God.

Paul too, before his conversion resisted the Holy Spirit. Eventually God knocked him off his horse.

> And when we had all fallen to the ground, I heard a voice saying to me in the Hebrew language, "Saul, Saul, why are you persecuting me? It is hard for you to kick against the goads." *Acts 26:14 ESV*

God had been goading him—poking him as a farmer would poke an animal with a stick to get it moving in the right direction. Paul had been refusing to comply. Instead of submitting to the Prince of Peace, Paul had been lashing out against the pricks of the Holy Spirit, and, as Jesus points out, life is hard when you kick against the goads.

It is indeed hard for the person who chooses not to be led by the Holy Spirit. For those folks, life is a continual battle between the will to do right and the desires of flesh. The will chooses to obey the laws dictated by their mind, but the flesh would rather go its own way. There is no victory for the believer living this way, relying on will power. It is only in surrender to the living God that we overcome.

> For if you live according to the flesh you will die, but if by the Spirit you put to death the deeds of the body, you will live. For all who are led by the Spirit of God are sons of God.
>
> *Romans 8:13 ESV*

RED CABBAGE

AGE 20.   It's the summer before my junior year in college, before the anorexia has fully taken root. I hitchhike up the West Coast USA with my friend Ann. It was a very unwise thing to do, but I was very unwise, and hitchhiking was safer then. A friendly young guy on summer break graciously offers to take us the whole distance.

Outside Eugene, Oregon, another hitchhiker climbs in, and it turns out to be an intensely good-looking young man my age whose name I have since forgotten. The young man asks to stop at the grocery store so he can get something to eat. He comes back to the car chomping with gusto on a head of red cabbage. Not a package of Twinkies. Not a bag of potato chips.   A head of red cabbage.   And he's enjoying it. I think, "Wow. This guy has control of appetite.   Who would eat raw red cabbage by choice?"

It's sunset when we arrive at his house, and this same incredibly peaceful, gentle, handsome guy gives us all permission to camp on the property. I don't want to sleep outside, and turn on my seductive spirit, but somehow he seems oblivious to it. Rarely if ever have I known this demonic influence not to work. My friend, Ann, who is beautiful and more wholesome than I, tries her wily innocence to attract him, but he isn't buying her flirtations either. He keeps talking about somebody he loves. It sounds like he's talking about a guy—and then I realize it's a dead guy. It finally dawns on me that he's talking about Jesus, and he's talking about Him like he loves Him. Could he really love God more than worldly pleasures?

The thought strikes both Ann and I like a rush of ice water. Neither of us has any more desire to travel. We abandon our hitchhiking, scrape the last of our money together, and fly home.

A man who had control over lusts. The idea shook me to the core.

> For everything created by God is good, and nothing is to be rejected if it is received with thanksgiving, for it is made holy by the word of God and prayer.   *I Timothy 4:4 ESV*

Paul wrote this to warn Timothy against those who promote abstinence from certain foods, foods that God created to be received with thanksgiving. But don't run off and buy a carton of Pop Tarts just yet. Yes, whatever is created by God is good, but there's food… and then there's food.

The book of Daniel teaches a good lesson about food. King Nebuchadnezzar assigned Daniel and his friends rations from his own table, and what did they do? They asked for vegetables instead. Nothing fancy, please. When the king's steward worried that vegetables wouldn't keep the young men strong, Daniel suggested a test.

> "Test your servants for ten days; let us be given vegetables to eat and water to drink. Then let our appearance and the appearance of the youths who eat the king's food be observed by you, and deal with your servants according to what you see."

> At the end of the ten days Daniel and his friends looked healthier and better nourished than any of the young men who ate the royal

food. So the guard took away their expensive food and the wine they were to drink and gave them vegetables instead.   *Daniel 1:12 ESV*

Healthier and better nourished. This is your Bible speaking.

Wise Solomon had advised centuries earlier:

When you sit down to eat with a ruler, observe carefully what is before you, and put a knife to your throat if you are given to appetite. Do not desire his delicacies, for they are deceptive food.   *Proverbs 23:1 ESV*

Deceptive food. Today in America we have king's food at our disposal all the time: refined flour, refined sugar, and a zillion even more highly refined products, some developed in laboratories. Do you read the ingredient labels of the foods you buy? Ignorance is not in your best interest.

My people are destroyed for lack of knowledge.   *Hosea 4:6 ESV*

Synthetically-processed foods have the taste that "all is well" when actually they are devoid of the life-giving forces that make food food. God put food together in whole packages perfectly designed for our health. Good natural food tastes better which means it is more satisfying. Good wholesome food contains the vital nutrients your body needs to have a wonderful day.

Your mood, your energy level, your outlook, are all affected by the nutrients you eat.

The Bible does not say you must not eat the king's treats, but it warns they are deceptive: deceptively pretty, deceptively luscious, and deceptively low in nutrients. The king's delicacies will titillate your tongue, but are of limited value for the rest of your body. In fact, most of the fancy processed foods will leave you feeling sluggish, nervous, anxious, and intensely desirous of more.

It is true, as it always has been, that everything created by God is good. If we choose according to His Spirit, we will be well fed.

If you're willing and obedient, you'll eat the best that the land produces. *Isaiah 1:19 ESV*

Perhaps you are afraid you can't afford to eat real, wholesome food. Yes, the fake foods are cheaper. But that which passes for food and is not food contains hidden medical dental costs that far exceed the price you pay for equivalent wholesome food. Your body is the temple of the Holy Spirit. What kind of temple should that be?

Our omniscient Creator is so wonderfully generous and caring. One of the many names for God in the Bible is *Yahweh Yireh*, meaning, "The Lord Will Provide." God cares for us with an eternal and everlasting love. Choose wisely, for you belong to Him.

MY SHEEP HEAR MY VOICE

AGE 20. Two weeks before college resumes, and I'm wallowing in emptiness. My parents have moved from the farm to northern New Jersey. The air is grey. I wander the suburbs for hours, trying to connect with something beyond myself that I am only half sure exists, and I come back feeling as hollow as I left.

I sit around trying to meditate, looking for life from books on Eastern religion, until finally my parents suggest I go to a commune in New Hampshire. They say it will be better than sitting around home.

The atmosphere at the commune seems good for seekers. We rise in the dark and watch in silence as the sun rises. Graceful stretching follows, then long solitary walks. It is on one of these walks, as I crest a high hill, that I suddenly remember something.

Hold it! Hold everything! I remember now. As a child I heard from the great Whoever! I don't remember what I heard, but I remember I was in bed and a heavenly voice comforted me. Nowhere in Buddhism or Taoism have I read that anyone could actually connect with the Great Whomever, and I did. It's possible!   I practically fly down the hill to the commune, tell them I'm quitting, and leave the next day.

THE FURNACE ROOM

AGE 20.   I'm late getting back to college, and end up renting an oversized closet in the bleak basement of an otherwise decent house on Grove Street. I am told the house rule is that everyone contributes equally to rent, but since my furnace room isn't really the equivalent of a room, I can eat any of the occupants' food for free. Weird arrangement. It doesn't work.

Because of course I feel uncomfortable about eating their food. And when I do get up my nerve to eat somebody's crackers, I overhear an annoyed voice asking, "Do you know who ate my crackers?" This happens more than once. And so I choose not to eat. It is good for me not to eat, I reason. Buddha is said to have survived on one grain of rice a day. So mostly I do without.

I know I need to eat, but I never lived off campus before. I don't know how to spend money, or budget, or buy groceries, or cook. I don't even know where the grocery store is.

Gradually the stress on my body takes its toll. The people in the house begin begging me to eat, but I tell them I am full. Sometimes I double up in pain from I know not what, probably a vitamin deficiency. I am too weak to open the heavy doors on campus. I faint in the women's locker room.

College seems stifling, a distraction. Within two weeks of my return to college, I drop out, overwhelmed with the shallowness of my life, the insufficiency of myself, and the inability of the world to do anything to help me. I have come to realize that my every thought is wretchedly self serving. Leaving behind boys and drugs and everything else that seems vain and frivolous, I begin to cry out to the Great Whomever, hoping to contact the Source of the Universe.

The cramps in my side that cause me to double over in pain increase. So I am walking down the sidewalk, aware that everything I have done to seek spiritual enlightenment has had the effect of shutting me out of society and destroying my health. Everything I have done to try to be more spiritual has made me fall further and further from the life I want.

Exploding with frustration, I turn to the heavenly Whoever and demand: "If I worked in Your factory, and I didn't know what I was supposed to do, or how I was supposed to do it, and yet I was always falling short, I would go on strike. So that's what I'm doing. I'm not going to try any more! I'm going on strike."

That's when I heard. The first time in years, maybe since childhood. And I heard...a sigh of relief. The

Eternal Source of the Universe responds with a very clear, very patient, sigh of relief.

What? He/she is glad I am giving up trying? He doesn't want me to do religious stuff?

How precious, that sigh! I can stop wearing robes? I don't need to empty my mind in boring meditation? I don't have to live a solitary existence on minimal food?

The relief washes over my soul. I have the ear of the Factory Owner of the Universe, and He wants me to quit trying.

CHAPTER 7
THE WAY

In this precious moment, as I have made contact with the Eternal and have His ear, I think, "What else can I ask?"

Okay, how about this? Please let me meet someone who can show me what you want me to do. How to live. An example. A model.

I know I've been heard. So hopeful, eager, and attentive, I keep my spiritual senses attuned to anyone the Great Spirit sends my way. Nothing happens. I go to bed, and the next day nothing happens. My attention is drawn to no person, and no one approaches me or even looks my way. In fact, it has been the most disappointing day of my life.

I begin to consider that even the master of the universe, the Great Whomever, has no true followers, and no genuine example to show me on Earth. My spirit feels like the polluted rain that drizzles down that chill November afternoon.

The streets are pretty much empty. Grove Street is deserted. My eyes are on the sidewalk, as I trudge home to my dreary furnace room. But as I get near home, suddenly I get an overwhelming feeling that if I look up right now, the person will be there.

I look up. Down a ways, there is someone. She's skipping and singing alone there in that dark gray chill drizzle of November. I have no idea how old she is, maybe seven. It's a little girl.

I had been hoping the person would be a nice-looking male my age. But a little child? You want me to become like a little child?

What a wonderful thought.

RESURRECTION

AGE 20. I awake suffocating under the weight of my sin. Stumbling up the basement stairs, I emerge in the morning light with my heart desperate to connect to the Source of Life. From the depths of my soul, I pour out a cry to the Creator of space and time,

Immediately I sense a presence, and recognize the same presence I experienced in nature in childhood—almost undetectable, but absolutely real. A deep voice echoes clearly inside my heart: "You have called to Me many times in the past, and each time I helped you. But each time after you received help, you turned and went your own way." I know what the voice says is true. Then I hear, "This is your last chance."

I see a clear vision of a vortex swirling downward, and know that it is the entrance to hell. Terrifyingly so. I am immediately reassured by this Presence that He wants to save me, if only I will abandon my life so He can. I see a list like a tickertape of what I need to give up to be saved. What they were, I can't remember, but I think there were seven...things like my plans for today and tomorrow, my idea of fun, my opinions on life, who my friends are, my future, my words.

I agree to do so. Immediately I feel a release. So this is salvation! I am overwhelmed, but before I have time to think, an invisible force draws me to follow after. It is very strong, but gentle and polite, so I allow myself to be led. I love adventure. But then I hesitate. I might faint on the way. I've been fainting lately, and I haven't eaten anything. Maybe I better turn back. The word "faith" comes to me. It's a word I never understood before. Now it becomes clear. I follow.

This firm but gentle pull continues to lead me (is it an angel?) and we arrive at a busy intersection. I know this place too well. The rush of cars has always frightened me. But today, tucked in next to this Spirit guide, I cross in perfect peace.

He/she/whatever takes me onward toward the women's gymnasium, where for the last two school-years I have spent so much time trying to swim away fat and guilt. But we don't stop there. We continue on to the M.S.U. library, and It pauses out front. There a tall fountain issues sparkling streams of water in the morning sun.

The Spirit pulls me onward, and as we enter the library, I am confronted by a milling mass of college students. Fear takes hold of me. I don't like crowds, and I especially don't want to be thought of as insane. I begin to thumb through a stack of magazines, pretending to act normal. Here is an interesting one, beautiful photos with natural food recipes…. Let's see. Add the…

Recipes??? I was led here by the eternal force of the universe and I want to read recipes? I throw down the magazine and seek after the strange Guide again.

It's no use. It's gone. There is no leading. No voice. I am alone again in a dark world without hope. Entering the stairwell, I cry out in desperation with only the slightest hope the invisible leading will return.

But there it is. This Spirit comes again, lifting my head and drawing me onward. There seems to be a principle here: Give up, and you will get help. Don't give up, no help. I hurry up the stairs after the Guide, who seems excited for me to follow.

We land on the third floor—I didn't even know this floor existed—and I follow my guide to a set of dimly-lit shelves near the back. No one is on this floor except me. Us.

My hand reaches toward a hardcover book on the top shelf. My mind is whirling. The book is green. Green is the color of healing in Buddhism. This book must be the work of a very great guru. I am amazed. In awe.

But the title—Good News—about knocks me to the floor. Who knew I needed good news more than I needed anything else in the world? Who knew? It's a book I've never heard of. Good News. My soul trembles as I open it. Before I look inside, a male voice thunders, absolutely thunders, in my right ear, louder than anything I have ever heard before:

I am the Way.

I tremble at my own insignificance in comparison. Who am I to be in the presence of the One who holds all Power? The Creator. My eyes focus on the page, and I see the same words exactly, "I am the Way."

> "**I am the Way**, the Truth and the Life. No one comes to the Father but by Me." *Jn 14:6*

There is no doubt. The God of the Universe has just spoken to me. I snap the book closed in fright.

Then I open it again, and these words ring out:

> Whatever you ask for in prayer, believe that you have received it, and it will be yours.
> *Matthew 21:22 ESV*

Whatever I ask for, if I believe, I'll receive it? Who would dare make such a promise? What book is this? ... so many numbers on each page. I thumb through it, and one name keeps popping up—the name of Jesus. it begins to dawn on me.   This is a Bible?

TEETERING ON THE BRINK

AGE 20. Clinging to this amazing book, I want to drop to my knees and sob and rejoice and cry out in wonder. But I can't get past the idea that this is a library, and so I am torn. I remain standing there in awe, unsure how to how to respond to this heaven-sent message, but filled with relief.

Gradually, as I quaver in indecision—wanting to worship, but not knowing how—worried about acting too strangely in the library, I begin to consider the fact that this is a Bible. Questions seep into my mind. Is this really for me? I begin to consider returning the book to the shelf.

 After what seems like ages wavering between extremes of joy and doubt, I reach up to put it back. The Bible is for old ladies. It's meant to sit on a shelf and collect dust. The Bible is the antithesis of what I want for an answer. I am too cool, much too open-minded for outdated religion.

Yet my desperate condition causes me to pause and reexamine my choices. I can believe this book that appeared to me so miraculously so wonderfully, or I can reject it and forget the whole thing.

Okay, wait. Analyze the situation. Well, I know "a stitch in time saves nine." It has pretty much always held true. Hmmm.

Doesn't apply.

How about, "A bird in hand is worth two in the bush?" I do have the Bible in hand.

No, doesn't seem to apply.

Well, "Don't look a gift horse in the mouth." A horse's teeth grow as it ages. Don't look a gift horse in the mouth. Just accept the gift.

Oh. If this is God's gift to me.... Who am I to criticize this gift from God? My life is broken and irreparable. I would be foolish to reject it.

 Thank you God, thank you Jesus, for this book. I receive it as your gift. A tremendous relief overcomes me, a relief which has not left me to this day.

JUST LOOKING AT HIM WE ARE CHANGED

How can we follow the Spirit? How can we ever know His leading? God made it simple. Do we want to follow Christ? Set our eyes on Him.

The eye is the lamp of the body. So, if your eye is healthy, your whole body will be full of light, but if your eye is bad, your whole body will be full of darkness. *Mat. 6:22 ESV*

Tuck this verse away in your heart. If your eyes are set on Christ, your whole body will be full of light. And the wonderful results you will find when you try this in your kitchen! The eye set on Christ will always lead you right. Guaranteed. The eye set on this food or that food or this show or anything worldly will lead you off. (Lord, remind us again and again to set our eyes on You.) It doesn't mean we can't watch something or even look at food. It means look at whatever we're looking at through the clear lens of Christ.

Fixing our eyes on Jesus, the author and perfecter of faith. *Hebrews 12:2 NAS*

Try it now. Fix your eyes on Jesus and keep them there. Let no word come from your mouth that distracts your heart from communion with God. Let nothing interfere with your fellowship with God. Hold fast to the risen One, and He will hold fast to you. Now watch how this relationship changes you. Watch how your mind and thoughts move to a higher level than before, how your words edify, how your joy remains full. Watch how God's love flows through you. How blessed our Savior. Just looking at Him we are changed!

> Beloved, we are God's children now, and what we will be has not yet appeared; but we know that when He appears we shall be like Him, because we shall see Him as He is.
>
> *I John 3:2 ESV*

God is Spirit, translucent and transparent. You will be able to see more clearly with your eyes on Him. You will begin to see with the heart and mind of God. You will be able to order at a restaurant, pick the right clothes, make decisions that used to confound you, and you will find that those choices are easy, because the Holy Spirit is guiding you. Jesus is our example:

> "The Son can do nothing of His own accord, but only what He sees the Father doing. For whatever the Father does, that the Son does likewise.
>
> *John 5:19 ESV*

Even Jesus was wholly submitted to His Father in this way. As we stay immersed in His Love, open to His leading, looking to Him and Him alone, we will walk in His peace, His joy, His love all the day long.

> I have set the LORD always before me; because He is at my right hand, I shall not be shaken.
>
> *Psalm 16:8 ESV*

SHOUT IT FROM THE HOUSETOPS

The first dilemma of my believing life... I can't take the Bible home. I'm a college drop out, which means no more library card. Hmmm. As long as I return it.... In faith, I stuff the *Good News* under my sweater and head for the door. No alarm sounds. I'll return it when I get another Bible.

I emerge into the light of day, feeling absolutely new. In a moment my life changed from harried, fretful, lost to accepted, loved, cherished by the Great Whomever. I have great peace and joy in the newfound Spirit.

Outside the library, students are milling around, and I spot an old friend. I tell him confidently, "I've found it! I've found what we've been looking for! I've found reality!" All the while I'm thinking "Where did this boldness come from?"

"Jesus said, 'I am the Way, the Truth, and the Life. No one comes to the Father except by Me.'" Why am I speaking so loudly? People around us can hear me.

I know nothing of Jesus' command to go into all the world and share the good news. I just want to. Like if you found the solution to cancer you'd want to tell everybody. And in the telling, I feel my soul beginning to heal.

My friend amazes me by scoffing, "We went through that last year," as if it's a fad. I just walk on in the Spirit, eager to tell anyone and everyone what has happened, and Who the Master of the Universe Is.

On the street corner I sing loud, unembarrassed, "Jesus is the way! He is the truth! He is the Life!" The owner of the corner café invites me in. He offers me a free soft drink, but I decline and speak to the crowd gathered there of Jesus and the Bible and what happened. The owner is kind, but after awhile gets nervous about losing customers and asks me to leave.

I head down Grove Street toward home. Under the branches of an old tree, it occurs to me that I haven't apologized to the Great Whomever, who now has a name, for how I have wasted my life. "Jesus, I am so very sorry for how I have messed up the life You gave me." I begin to list my sins: "I've lived in lust...".

But before I can say another word, there comes a deep assurance that's it's all been wiped clean. I don't need to look back. I don't need to apologize any more. It is finished.

I see what must be a vision of a dark hillside, the cross, a person nailed to it. The eyes of Jesus look down at me kindly, and suddenly I see. He did it for me.

HOW DO I KNOW IT'S YOU, GOD?

How do we know we are being led by God? How did Jesus know He was being led by God when He called the Pharisees snakes and vipers? *(Mathew 23:33)* How did He know it was the Father's will for Him to turn the tables of the money-changers? *(Mathew 23:27)* How did King David decide it was okay to dance in his underclothes in public? *2 Samuel 6* How do we ever know for sure if the Holy Spirit is leading us? Listen to the words of Jesus:

> **If anyone's will is to do God's will, he will know whether the teaching is from God.**
> *John 7:17 ESV*

Jesus said we will know whether a teaching is from God if we are willing to do God's will. If we can know whether a teaching is from God, we will also know whether a leading is of God the same way, by our willingness to do His will. If we're willing, the Holy Spirit will lead us. As we submit wholly and humbly to His governance, the Lord God will guide us and empower us in His perfect will.

Wholly submitted, with your mind and heart on Christ, you will live in a gradually growing love relationship with Him. You will know the ever-present gentle nudges of the Holy Spirit: "This is the way, walk therein." Your life will be filled with a new certainty, and with a peace which passes all understanding.

CHAPTER 8
MORE POWER, MORE HOLY SPIRIT

> Peter and John... came down and prayed for them that they might receive the Holy Spirit, for he had not yet fallen on any of them, but they had only been baptized in the name of the Lord Jesus. Then they laid their hands on them and they received the Holy Spirit.
>
> Acts 8:14 ESV

AGE 21   In those first couple weeks, I go from a weak, malnourished 100 pounds to a healthy, energetic 135 pounds, and have stayed that way (plus or minus a few pounds) ever since. But temptations begin to surface. I know I've been born again, but spiritually I'm beginning to flounder. When I last opened the Bible, I read "Woe to you," and it scared me into not reading it any more. I keep hoping to meet someone who has come to know Jesus for real, but I don't have the slightest clue where to turn.

A year passes and I still haven't met anyone who talks about Christ! I decide to take matters into my own hands and begin searching. Catholics talk a lot about Jesus, I reason, so it seems like a good place to start. I have plenty of studying to do now that I'm re-enrolled in college, and I take a load of books to the Catholic church basement to study there. Hours go by, hoping someone will come along to talk to me about Jesus. Suddenly, two nuns approach, and I think I've hit the jackpot.

"Excuse me. I met Jesus, and I need to know a lot more about Him. Could you talk with me please?"

They seem distracted. "There is a class on Thursday nights at 6:30. The new classes start next week." Then they walk away.

That's it? If they knew the Jesus I know, they would've exploded with joy to talk about Him. But they didn't. Neither do the nice young people I sit next to when I go to mass that Sunday.

"Sorry. We really have too much homework to stay and talk about Jesus with you."

I begin to realize what a special gift I have. Faith isn't something you get just by going to church. I realize I need an extra dose of power if I'm going to live this Christian life in holiness. I begin to call out to God, honestly confessing my weakness. Before long I am rewarded.

I bump into an ex-hippie I knew from a new age psychology class I took before my encounter with

Christ. But the air of superiority this guy used to hold is now gone. He seems almost innocent, and he seems shiny. I explain to him that I found Jesus, and he bubbles with enthusiasm, and keeps saying, "Praise God! Praise God!"

I'm not sure why he's telling me to "Praise God!", especially since I don't hear him praising God, but I get the sure sense that the God I know is the God he knows. He invites me to a meeting that night. I accept.

They pick me up at home, and we park across from a house not far away. The street is dark and the traffic moves fast. As we cross, one of the young men gently holds my elbow. How did he know that I needed assurance?

Inside, there are maybe 12 college kids singing worship songs. I peek toward the kitchen, expecting to see an adult making Kool-Aid in there. None. These young people like me are worshipping, not to impress an adult, but because they want to. This is heavy.

A couple of them begin talking and I don't know what they're talking about, but I keep hearing the phrase, "baptism in the Holy Spirit." I ask, "How do you get baptized in the Holy Spirit?"

One of them, a girl with sand-colored hair (I think her name was Angel) tells me they are from the Glory Barn in Indiana and says to follow her. So as not to interfere with the worship, we go down the slim steps to the dim basement and there she opens the Bible. She shows me that Jesus commanded His followers to be baptized in water, to take communion in His remembrance, and to be baptized with the Holy Spirit.

> He ordered them not to depart from Jerusalem, but to wait for the promise of the Father, which, he said, "you heard from me; for John baptized with water, but you will be baptized with the Holy Spirit not many days from now."   Acts 1:5 ESV

She says the baptism of the Spirit is received through the laying on of hands, and the Spirit is given to those who obey. (Acts 5:32) I say, "Well, you know, I don't always obey. I want to, but I know I don't always." She says my honesty is good. That's why Jesus died for us. We must trust His righteousness, which is given to us freely at the cross, and not our own.

Then she shows me how the weak, wavering disciples were transformed into dynamic preachers by this baptism in the Holy Spirit. They received boldness to be Christ's witnesses even unto death.

And she shows me where the followers of Jesus spoke in tongues when they were Spirit baptized:

> All of them were filled with the Holy Spirit and began to speak in other tongues as the Spirit enabled them.   *Acts 2:4 NIV*

She questions me to be sure I'm ready—no unconfessed sin, no unforgiveness. She tells me to seek God deeply and earnestly in worship. She tells me to say "Hallelujah" over and over, keeping my eyes fixed on Jesus. Meanwhile, she will speak in tongues next to me. At some point, out of my mouth will flow words I don't recognize, and that is the Holy Spirit of God.

I do what she says, looking to the Lord and seeking Him in all His glory. And just as she said, it happens. I speak in an unknown tongue. At first it seems silly, strange, but as I continue for a few seconds I feel a release of my spirit! Like a plug has been pulled, my mouth gushes forth the unintelligible praises of God. I am filled with joy and wonder, and everything under my closed eyelids turns a heavenly bright, brighter than gold—so bright that finally I have to look away.

We pray together and give thanks, and then go upstairs. The meeting is ending, and they offer me a ride home. I decline politely, and run the few blocks home, running more freely than I have ever run. It seems like flying. At home, I sit on the edge of my bed and open the Bible. The words leap out at me. I can understand what I am reading! The scriptures that seemed so unintelligible before speak to me now as clearly as a child's book.

For the first time since I have given my life to Christ, I can read the Bible and understand it... and the words are sweeter to me than honey.

I remember thinking that, had I taken heed of even one short sentence of this book earlier in life, it would have saved me years of trouble.

Following Christ is like swimming. Children pretend to swim while their feet are still planted on the ground, and before Christ, we pretended to be good. Then one day we surrendered, and felt the water lift us from the world. No longer tied to its approval, we now live by faith. But that was just the beginning. There is so much more beneath the waves. Being born again was just the beginning. Being baptized in the Holy Spirit is to dive deep, to be fully immersed in Jesus.

THY KINGDOM COME

Jesus gave us this promise:

> Ask, and it will be given to you; seek, and you will find; knock, and it will be opened to you. For everyone who asks receives, and the one who seeks finds, and to the one who knocks it will be opened.
>
> *Luke 11:9 ESV*

The Greek word for "ask" is in the present active imperative tense. That means it doesn't just mean ask. It means "ask and keep on asking." The word for "seek" doesn't just mean "seek". It means "seek and keep on seeking." "Knock" means "Knock and keep on knocking."

And for what should we keep asking, seeking, knocking?

> What father among you, if his son asks for a fish, will instead of a fish give him a serpent; or if he asks for an egg, will give him a scorpion? If you then, who are evil, know how to give good gifts to your children, how much more will the heavenly Father give the Holy Spirit to those who ask Him!
>
> *Luke 11:10 ESV*

The Lord wants us to keep asking, seeking and knocking to receive the Holy Spirit. It is the Holy Spirit who will restore liberty to the captive soul. It is the Holy Spirit who will enable us to do the works that Jesus did, including healing the sick, casting out demons, and raising the dead.

Every ounce of God's Spirit is available to us, and it is His joy to give us the Holy Spirit! With the baptism of the Holy Spirit, we can operate in the kingdom of God in power!

> Do not seek what you are to eat and what you are to drink, nor be worried. For all the nations of the world seek after these things, and your Father knows that you need them. Instead, seek his kingdom, and these things will be added to you.
>
> *Luke 12:29 ESV*

THY WILL BE DONE

Most people with eating problems set themselves up for failure at the grocery store. Buying something without nutritional benefit simply because it tantalizes your taste buds is inviting a battle once you get home.

For me, it was cookies. Like me, maybe, you know you won't eat just one, or two, or six, or eight. Those cookies will keep drawing you, and you will have to keep resisting and resisting and resisting until you finally decide it's easier just to eat the whole bag.

> But put on the Lord Jesus Christ, and make no provision for the flesh, to gratify its desires. *Romans 13:14 ESV*

No provision for the flesh. That means not buying food that will tempt you. Is it worth the fight against temptation once you get home? If you are addicted to it—don't buy it. Sell all that you have for that pearl of great price. Sell all that you have for God's purity, and the glorious peace that comes with obedience.

You are making life and death decisions every time you go to the grocery store. What you choose can mean the difference between a long, energetic life radiating God's goodness…and a depressed lethargic life that is cut short by illness. Giving the Lord your full attention as you shop will save you a week's worth of agonizing trouble trying to resist temptation when you get home. The Lord would love to lead you up and down each aisle.

When your eyes and heart are set on God, He will show you what to buy. I can guarantee, that is how Jesus shopped.

> **He will delight in the fear of the Lord, And He will not judge by what His eyes see, nor make a decision by what His ears hear.**
> *Isaiah 11:3 NAS*

Sometimes the Lord will lead you to read the ingredient label, and that can be shocking at times. You'll find that not all things sold in the name of food are really food. Any grocery item that is solely for your taste buds and not for your body is not food at all. The Lord will lead you away from buying addictive nonfoods, and will satisfy you far better with the rich nutrition of Garden of Eden food.

For years I had to avoid buying cookies because I knew I was addicted to them. I didn't want to give the devil an opportunity to harass me with temptation and guilt. So I learned, by the graceful leading of the Holy Spirit, to leave the too-tempting food on the shelf of the store where it belonged.

Gradually (and here's the wonderful part!) I lost a taste for such things. They lost their appeal. You could wave a chocolate chip cookie or fudge brownie under my nose and I would only be mildly interested. I have come to understand the value of real food. When I want something to eat, I look for what I call real food.

With your mind set on Jesus, He'll show you how to compare prices. But He won't always lead you to the cheapest. Buying the healthiest food you can buy is a lot cheaper than paying the medical bills that result from poor nutrition.

Jesus's gentle leading will give you wisdom as you look to Him every step of the way. And do! For you will find that the bags of groceries you bring home are infinitely more satisfying than what you would have picked out without Him. You'll be able to eat food you prepare at home with your own hands, knowing that the ingredients are clean and wholesome. You will feast and enjoy true liberty throughout the week. Your meals will be tastier, your health will improve, and your heart will abound in thanksgiving toward God.

Win the war at the grocery store, and when you get home you will fight no more.

SHOPPING IN THE SPIRIT

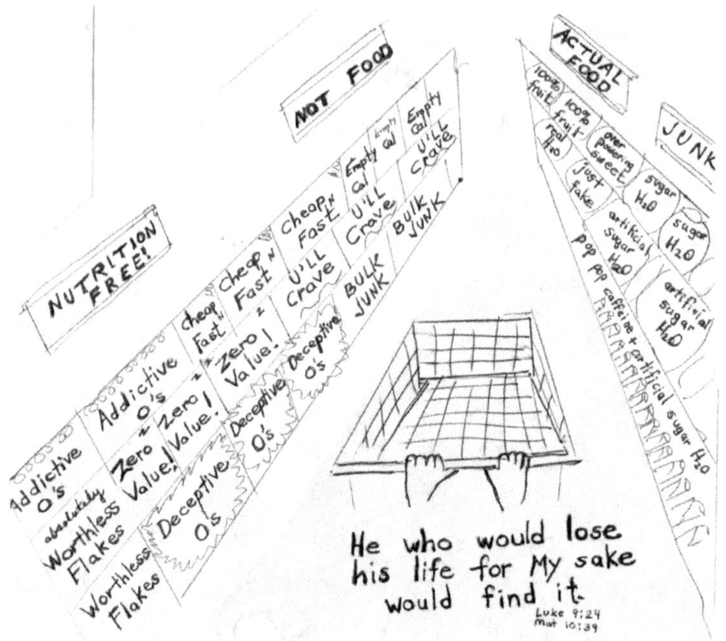

To be led by the Spirit. It is the end of striving. It is to enter into an eternal rest. To rest is to cease from trying. To let Him lead is to be as a child in your daddy's arms, floating on water. Daddy's got you. And what wonderful adventures He has for you!

AGE 21: I was a new Christian, recently baptized in the Spirit, I lived off campus, and had to do my own grocery shopping. Money was short; it was critical that I make wise choices. I needed direction to buy food that would taste good, satisfy, and keep me healthy. And I needed His wisdom to somehow stretch a tiny bit of money across the whole week. In this matter I had no choice but to completely let go and let God lead. It was a scary proposition, but I knew there was no other way. Would I let myself be led by this Holy Spirit in the grocery aisles, His unseen Hand guiding me I knew not where?

My old nature would never have allowed it. I had basically never allowed my body to be led by a spiritual force until I met Jesus, and certainly never in a grocery store. But here I was, fixing my eye on Christ, leaning on the Spirit of God, bending my ear to hear, waiting for the gentle tug on my body that would indicate "this way" and then waiting for the pull on my hand to reach for whatever the Holy Spirit indicated.

I was not disappointed.

> Hope does not disappoint.
>
> *Romans 5:5 NAS*

When your hope is set in the Lord, you will never be disappointed. I didn't know that then. I just hoped if I put the reins in God's hands I would get some sense of what to buy. Ah, it was better than I had anticipated. Not only did God give me general ideas about what to eat, and whatnot, He specifically led my hand to this product and that. It was years ago, but I remember distinctly He led me to the fish.

I had never cooked fish in my life. I had never really cooked much of anything on a stove in my life. I had no idea how to cook it, but the leading was very strong, so I ignored the sense of revulsion I felt at picking up this scaly creature with an eye, and put it in my basket.

I remember having the most wonderful dinner that night of poached fish with a plateful of brown rice and maybe some coleslaw, followed by herb tea. I remember feeling perfectly full, absolutely satisfied, and very happy. It was a brand new feeling.

Where was the craving for dessert, I wondered? It never happened.

Still under the leading of the Holy Spirit, I took a shower, and was led to run my fingernails under the powerful stream of water. Then I sat down with a glass of water (something new for me) to study, and realized for the first time in years I wasn't biting my fingernails. Later in the evening I had some more chamomile tea and slept peacefully, without any of the wild, tortured, dreams that had been my norm.

It was possible! Health was on its way. All glory to the Living God!

GOD IS NOT PUSHY

> If you live according to the flesh you will
> die, but if by the Spirit you put to death
> the deeds of the body, you will live. For
> all who are led by the Spirit of God are
> sons of God. *Romans 8:12 ESV*

All who are led by the Spirit of God are sons of God. But how do we know it's God? Is it a voice? Not usually. The Lord God will speak through an inner voice, but more often through a gentle tug. He does not push. That is key. The Holy Spirit, who came down from heaven as a dove and rested upon Jesus *(Matthew 3:16)*, is gentle and lowly and kind. The Holy Spirit is not pushy. If you feel pressured to do something, look to Christ for direction. The Holy Spirit does not demand His own way *(I Corinthians 13)*; He gently guides.

When God does speak words to me, it is most often in a gentle whisper. *(I Kings 19:11)* Sometimes my mind can hear it. Sometimes only my heart can sense it. Don't expect God to speak as loud as your phone or your friend. God does not need to shout, but for those who listen, his voice is discernable.

AGE 21. I was newly baptized in the Spirit, and by golly, I wanted to be spiritual. Or maybe I just wanted to be considered spiritual. Not understanding the generous grace of God, and the fact that He alone could save me, I thought it my duty to press in hard no matter what. I prayed long hours on my knees, and despite increasing fatigue and fading health, stayed up later and later each night, influenced by voices: "Get down on your knees", "Pray longer," "That's not enough. Pray more."

I didn't know it, but instead of being led by God, I was being influenced by a spirit of religiosity whose desire was to wear me down, causing me to stay up late and rise early to pray, day after day after day. This wearing down left me vulnerable to even more trouble, as I finally suspected when it began to lead me to walk across busy streets without checking for cars. This was not good.

Fortunately, I shared my concern with some good believing friends, who convinced me that the Spirit of God is always peaceful and open to reason.

> The wisdom from above is first pure, then peaceable, gentle, open to reason, full of mercy and good fruits, impartial and sincere.
>
> *James 3:1 ESV*

They exhorted me to stop listening to the spirit I was hearing. I objected, wanting to be holy, wanting to please God. I was honest with them—I didn't dare to stop listening to the voices.

They responded, "If God wants to talk to you, don't you think He can do so whether you are listening or not?" And that, I acknowledged, was true.

So I stopped listening to the voices, and immediately found rest and peace. God still spoke to me, and I to Him, but the deluding, demanding voices were gone. Praise God! Praise God for friends in the Body of Christ who were walking in the Spirit and had the mind of the Spirit to save me from delusion!

So walk in the Spirit, and in so doing, be grateful for and cultivate relationships with those who seek God earnestly. I know now the inner voice of the Holy Spirit is one of peace. His gentle leading is peaceful.

Even when the Holy Spirit convicts of sin His voice is peaceful and full of mercy.

Satan would like to lead you around like a pig with a ring in its nose.

Jesus is the Good Shepherd. You know His voice. Follow Him.

Satan is the one with the pitchfork.

FROM THE HAND OF GOD

We can learn from the animals in the wild, whose bodies glorify God. Look at the supreme beauty exhibited by each one. They do not strive to be thin, and none are overweight. Deer eat corn from our fields as much as they want whenever they want, and they can still leap over the fence and run like the wind. Birds don't overeat at our feeders. Wild animals know how to eat.

> I tell you, do not be anxious about your life, what you will eat or what you will drink, nor about your body, what you will put on. Is not life more than food, and the body more than clothing? Look at the birds of the air: they neither sow nor reap nor gather into barns, and yet your heavenly Father feeds them. Are you not of more value than they?
>
> *Matthew 6:25 ESV*

Yet for many of us, there is a tendency to eat whatever we can while we can. Perhaps we have faced food insecurity at some time in our lives. When there's food in front of us, we think we'd better eat it while we can, storing up for when we can't. But the belly is not a good place to store food. It's designed to take in just enough for what we need, nothing more. Our Heavenly Father cherishes the wild animals and provides for them as He provides for us. For them, so for us—His grace is entirely sufficient.

AGE 21. Still a new believer, I was unemployed and hungry. I knew nothing about applying for food stamps, and my cupboards dwindled to only the previous tenant's macaroni and powdered milk. Have you ever tried to live solely off macaroni and powdered milk for a week?

After a couple days, your body can't take any more of it. My kindhearted landlady must have gotten wind that my cupboards were bare, because she began offering me odd jobs every day, sewing a curtain hem, mending a rug, so that I had a couple dollars to buy a nutrition bar or an apple. And then my future husband must have recognized the sorry state I was in, because he asked me to marry him! God is so good.

Still, there were times in marriage where money ran down and dwindled, even while I was nursing one child and putting food on the table for two others. God did not depart from us, but gave us through this a great sense of appreciation for food. To this day, I love to go grocery shopping, and marvel at the wonders available to us in the store. This thankfulness for food is a wonderful gift, and I feel sorry for those who complain about having to grocery shop, people who I guess have never experienced the Lord meeting their need a day at a time in wonderful ways.

CHAPTER 9
THE HEART'S DELIGHT

Delight yourself in the Lord, and He
will give you the desires of your heart.

Psalm 37:4 ESV

Such good news. If we delight ourselves in the Lord, we receive our heart's desire. Then again, if our heart's desire is to eat a dozen doughnuts, it is likely we are not delighting ourselves in the Lord. If our heart's desire is to look sexy in a bathing suit, we are most likely not delighting ourselves in the Lord. If our heart's desire is to be skinnier than our friends, we are likely not delighting ourselves in the Lord. When we delight ourselves in the Lord, our desire is for a healthy body that glorifies Jesus, holy and blameless. And isn't that what we really want?

When we delight ourselves in the Lord—who He is and what He is doing—we will see our dreams come true.

No good thing does He withhold from those who walk uprightly. *Psalm 84:11 ESV*

Our Heavenly Father will abundantly fulfill the good desires while helping us abandon the worthless ones. The worthless stuff you thought you needed will become unnecessary, and the really good stuff will suddenly be exactly what you want.

GUARD YOUR HEART

No surprise: Satan is working hard to undermine your faith, and one of his favorite tools is discouragement. If the Devil can make you look bad to yourself—if he can get you to think there is no way out of your predicament—then his quest to steal, kill, and destroy your faith becomes a lot easier.

One of Satan's main ploys is to confuse you into thinking you are fat forever—that God really can't (and won't ever) lead you into a healthy relationship with food and a healthy body. Like Eve in the Garden of Eden, we hear the Devil whisper, "Has God said?"

The enemy loves nothing more than to stealthily ease your mind off Christ, and get you obsessing about food. He begins sweetly, so sweetly that you will not be aware of the fact that his plan is to head you downward into a cycle of ever-deepening depression. Once Satan gets a toehold, he can begin to wear you down with guilt and accusations, and with resolutions that he knows will ultimately fail. The Devil has rendered us ineffective for the Kingdom of God every time he succeeds in getting our minds off Christ.

There's no time to pray, no desire to worship, no thought to sing praise, no giving of thanks when a believer is absorbed in what he should or should not have eaten.

And all the while, Christ looks on your heart.

Man looks on the outward appearance, but the Lord looks on the heart. *I Sam 16:7*

If your heart is right with God, so will your mind be. If your mind is right with God, so will your eye be. If your eye is right with God, so will your actions be. And if your actions are right with God, so will your body be. It is all hinged together, and it begins with a heart steadfastly devoted to God.

Above all else, guard your heart, for everything you do flows from it. *Prov. 4:23 NIV*

How often do you get on the scale to see what you weigh? And what's the point? Is worry going to erase an inch from your waistline? Does worry work? Has it worked so far? I don't own a scale. Why bother?

Jesus said, "Apart from Me you can do nothing."

Apart from Me you can do nothing.
John 15:5 ESV

Remember those words. Meditate on them. They are life to your soul. And don't worry about the Devil.

The devil who deceived them was thrown into the lake of fire and brimstone...and will be tormented day and night forever and ever. *Revelation 20:10 NAS*

Yahoooooo!

THIS THING CALLED PRAYER

> ...praying at all times in the Spirit, with all prayer and supplication.
>
> *Ephesians 6:18 ESV*

Prayer is a great privilege. We can pray for wisdom at the grocery store. We can pray for guidance as we cook. We can pray that we learn to like vegetables. We can pray for understanding. We can pray that we get enough sleep. We can pray with the author of Proverbs:

> Feed me with the food that is my portion, that I not be full and deny You and say, "Who is the Lord?" Or that I not be in want and steal, and profane the name of my God.
>
> *Proverbs 30:9 NAS*

God loves honest prayer.

I often pray, "Help me God to want to do your will."

And if I'm not sure about something I pray, "Lord, convince me if this is your will."   He does.

Jesus—God in human form—cried out to His Father:

> In the days of His flesh, Jesus offered up prayers and supplications, with loud cries and tears, to Him who was able to save Him from death, and He was heard because of His reverence.   *Hebrews 5:7 ESV*

Even the very Son of God while on Earth felt the need to pray, and to pray with loud cries and tears. So we need to pour out our hearts to God. On a walk, in the bathroom, in the car, in bed, every time we are alone—wherever we are—what a joy to pour out our hearts to God.

We ask once, and we keep on asking, believing for the answer. We knock once, and we keep on knocking until the answer is revealed. We seek the Lord's face, and we keep on seeking because He loves us. As we draw near, the Father draws near to us. He will whisper in our ears that we are not forgotten, that He loves us with an everlasting love. And He will give us the keys to life.

ZING!

Looking at me, you would not have known that my life once revolved completely around food and what others thought of me. But, even years after I was born again, a good portion of my thoughts went like this:

"Should I have eaten that? I wish I didn't. Why did I eat that? It really wasn't worth it. Why did I eat so much? How can I stop? What do I need to do to be slim?" ... and on and on.

What a shameful waste of mental space, don't you agree? By all means buy the freshest, healthiest food that is available to you. But remember, it's not about food. Jesus said:

> It is not what goes into the mouth that defiles a person, but what comes out of the mouth; this defiles a person...Do you not see that whatever goes into the mouth passes into the stomach and is expelled? But what comes out of the mouth proceeds from the heart, and this defiles a person.
>
> *Matthew 15:11 ESV*

So it's not what you eat; it's what you think and say that matters. Every decision we make is an eternal one. We place our trust in Christ to serve and obey Him, or we choose to turn away and go off on our own. Our mindset today determines our future, both in this life and the next:

Paul tells us to hold every thought up to Christ.

> **We...take every thought captive to obey Christ.**
>
> *II Corinthians 10:5 ESV*

It works something like this. Eyes see cream-filled doughnut. Subconscious mind thinks: My family ate doughnuts with cream inside. I miss my family. That cream-filled doughnut will make me happy. I should eat it now right now before anything stops me.

But first, we check with the Lord. Zing...we send the thought to Christ. He catches it and in my heart I instantly see that the doughnut will never satisfy that longing for family, nor will its empty calories satisfy my stomach. I am instantly convinced, and I no longer want the dumb doughnut.

In making the decision to look to Him, to seek His advice, I instantly find peace. The dread that I might lose out on something special, and fear I might not get to eat it is gone! I am free! What a happy day! Christ knows I love the idea of those doughnuts, but I now know I can live without one. In fact, I can live more peacefully without one.

Praise God! I am free! I love being free! If my mind wanders back to the doughnut—now the jelly one has caught my eye—I cast that thought upon the Lord as well. I remember that I am free to do all things in Christ, so I let Him lead. A couple burritos, some coleslaw, an apple. I walk away perfectly satisfied. More satisfied than I would ever be with powdered sugar on the end of my nose.

THE MIND AT REST

It is so easy to think it is not important what we think about. Yet Jesus rebuked Peter for his worldly thinking:

> "Get behind me, Satan! You are a hindrance to me. For you are not setting your mind on the things of God, but on the things of man." *Matthew 16:23 ESV*

The rebuke is for me. How often do I find myself focusing on my problems, on my circumstances, on my opinions, my desires, without letting God in on the conversation? How often do I focus on something instead of God, and rush off after that thing that God is not leading me to. Idols. When I focus on this world I am not being changed into Christ's likeness, I am not reflecting His glory, I am not showing His love, and I have become a hindrance to God's kingdom on earth.

So we need to stay focused on Christ. But take heed: You don't need to tell your mind to worship Christ. Just let it. You don't need to nag your spirit to praise the Lord. Give it the freedom to do so. For this your mind was created. For this your spirit was given. It is God's will that you are in Christ Jesus. He chose you and loved you before you ever thought to turn His way. And now nothing can separate you from His love, not any power on earth or heaven.

We won't ever run out of things to think about with our minds resting on the love of God. God is love. And love is the magnet that holds us to Him.

> **God is love, and whoever abides in love abides in God, and God abides in him.**
>
> *I John 4:16 ESV*

God Is Love. Let it be known to every living soul: God Is Love. Let it be known to the cell phone representative who has left you on hold: God Is Love. Let it be known to the children when they refuse to obey. God Is Love Let it be known to the teenager tailgating your car. God Is Love. Let it be known to the neighbor who lets his dog poop on your lawn. God Is Love. Let it be known to everyone who would frazzle you and degrade you and harass you for their own selfish pleasure. God is love.

Oh, Lord, teach us this simple truth.

EVERY THOUGHT

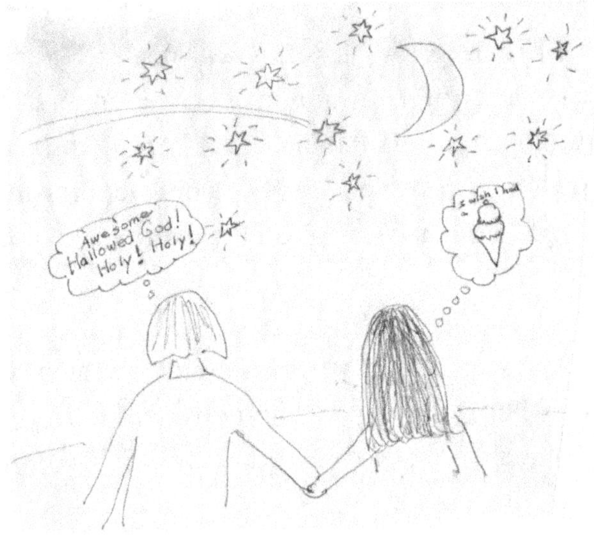

Casting down imaginations, and every high thing that exalteth itself against the knowledge of God, and bringing into captivity every thought to the obedience of Christ.   *II Corinthians 10:5 KJV*

Every thought? When I first read that, all I could think was "impossible." But I'm finding that taking every thought captive to Christ isn't as hard as it sounds. It's a resting of the mind in the place of soothing tranquility which He offers.

Rejoice always, pray without ceasing, give thanks in all circumstances; for this is the will of God in Christ Jesus for you.

I Thessalonians 5:17 ESV

Pray without ceasing. Can we do that? Of course we can. And what great blessings will result! God doesn't want us chattering away at Him all day long, but He does want us to tune into His presence throughout the day, recognizing His presence right beside you, blessing Him, thanking Him, and passing to Him every need, your own and others'.

What a blessing we have to be able to rest our weary minds in Him abiding in His continual comfort, wise counsel, and perfect love. And don't think you need to pray long prayers.

> Guard your steps when you go to the house of God. To draw near to listen is better than to offer the sacrifice of fools, for they do not know that they are doing evil.

Ecclesiastes 5:1 ESV

Sometimes I hear people pray about every little thing on their mind, and I wonder: Are they interested at all in God's mind? Prayer to them must seem to be a burdensome chore, if they think they have to advise God about every little thing in their life.

Think of a surfer. She doesn't go out into the waves just to paddle and paddle and paddle around. No. She paddles out expectantly waiting for the wave to uplift and carry her. That's what happens when we paddle out to Him with holy reverence, thankful hearts, and a willingness to listen.

And when you pray, do not heap up empty phrases as the Gentiles do, for they think that they will be heard for their many words. Do not be like them, for your Father knows what you need before you ask Him.

Matthew 6:7 ESV

I have learned to begin my day acknowledging the Father and Son. Before I get dressed, before I eat breakfast, before I get out of bed, I seek the Lord in the Word. It seems to me He is never so near as He is when I first awaken.

I love them that love me; and those that seek me early shall find me. *Proverbs 8:17 KJV*

And it very much helps that I don't watch or listen to or read anything before I go to bed that could still be clouding my thoughts in the morning.

Equally significant, I make it a practice to seek God in Scripture before turning out the light next to my bed at night. You do have a light next to your bed, don't you? If you don't…get one, and keep your Bible there right where you can commune with God in His Word before sleep. Let him lead you where to open it and read until you hear his voice. That's what I do. A little night-night kiss from the Son. You will sleep with the peace of Jesus, and arise to seek Him fresh again.

WHY WOULD GOD WANT PRAISE?

> Let everything that has breath praise the Lord! Praise the Lord! *Psalm 150:6 ESV*

For many years I found it disconcerting to think that God would want us to praise Him. How could a God of humility want praise? An earthly person who demanded praise would be a megalomaniac, obsessed with power. If God is humble—as Jesus showed us He obviously is, healing the lepers, washing the disciples' feet, riding on a donkey, and dying in our place—why does He want our praise?

I struggled with the question for some time, until I finally got around to asking the Lord. Suddenly it dawned on me. He seeks our worship not for His sake, but for our sake. It is only through the heartfelt acknowledgement of Who God is that we can receive from Him all that He wants to give us.

> Nor is He served by human hands, as though He needed anything, since He Himself gives to all mankind life and breath and everything. *Acts 17:25 ESV*

We need to recognize how astoundingly wonderful God is. He is Eternal, Magnificent, High above all the Heavens. He puts His love in our hearts. Praise simply acknowledges Who He is!

Think of a solar collector. As a solar collector must be aligned to the sun in order to receive its energy, so praise aligns us to God. And our worship is a sweet aroma to YHWH.

Hallowed Father! Blessed Savior! Two hundred plus times in the Bible we are told to praise the Lord, and what a blessing it is to do so.

In heaven we will be so overcome with the realization of Who He Is that I'm guessing we will not be able to say anything except "Wow!" in all its many forms. We will say it for all eternity and still not have fully proclaimed His greatness! Hallelujah!

HIS OVERCOMING POWER

Jesus faced the most powerful temptations anyone could ever face, and the first one had to do with food. Jesus hadn't eaten for more than a month, and He was hungry. Who should show up at that very moment but the enemy of our souls to tempt Him?

> "If you are the Son of God, command these stones to become loaves of bread."
> *Matthew 4:3 ESV*

Even though He was ravenously hungry, Jesus knew this was not His Father speaking. So how did He respond to this frontal attack from Satan? Jesus called upon the Word…the Word He had hidden in his heart for just such a time as this. Jesus answered:

> "It is written, 'Man shall not live by bread alone, but by every word that comes from the mouth of God.'"
> *Matthew 4:4 ESV*

Jesus spoke directly to the devil with the Truth of God's Word. And that little sentence spoken confidently in submission to the Father did the trick. The temptation was over. Satan withdrew. Angels came and ministered to Jesus.

Satan can't get around the wall of faith you set up when you believe and trust whole-heartedly in the Word of God.

"Man shall not live by bread alone, but by every word that comes from the mouth of God...You shall not put the Lord your God to the test...You shall worship the Lord your God, and serve Him only." Three quick blows with the Word of God and Satan gave up tempting Him. The same defense that worked for Jesus will work for you when you encounter temptation. When Satan comes in like a flood, you will raise up a standard against him. Say whatever Scripture comes to mind, and say it loud and with utter confidence. Shout the Word, sing the Word, and stand on the Word of God.

Confidently confessing God's Word will purify your heart and send Satan running, in the same way that turning over a log and exposing it to the light sends the creeping things under it scurrying for cover. This is the power of the Word of God.

PRAISE THE LORD (let it pour)

Do your prayers seem flat? Does it seem like maybe He's not listening? Take this hint from the Word of God.

> **Enter His gates with thanksgiving, and His courts with praise!** *Psalm 100:4 ESV*

Praise flows from the Holy Spirit in you. It's not something you need to work up. You don't need to memorize what to say. Open the gates of your heart and let it pour—everything you know to be true about God.

All that He is is praiseworthy: He is our deliverer! Our hope! Our salvation! The healer *(Psalm 103:3)!!* He alone is the giver of health, our counselor, the One who guides us in righteousness. He empowers us to obey His Word. He makes us clean! He is the rest for our souls. He is tender toward us. He is the One who gives us words of praise to let flow from our innermost being. Praise the omnipotent Creator! Praise Him, the gentle lover of our souls.

The extra good thing is that the act of praising and thanking God sinks the truth of Who He Is deep into our being. Thus we grow in faith.

Praise God that He is teaching us to praise Him!!!!

KEEPING IT REAL

I was cooking in the kitchen and routinely singing some kind of praise song when God whispered to my heart: "Remember, this is a love relationship." Oh! So sweetly to be convicted. God does not want duty-bound praises. He does not want robotic thank you's. God seeks our sincere affection, as a loving bridegroom rejoices in the adoring gaze of his young bride.

The only way we can return such love is by presenting ourselves wholly to Him: body, soul, mind and spirit.

> I urge you, brothers and sisters, in view of God's mercy, to offer your bodies as a living sacrifice, holy and pleasing to God—this is your true and proper worship.
>
> *Romans 12:1 NIV*

When we give ourselves to Him, He shows Himself to us. Then it is only natural to acknowledge His goodness, His mercy, His sustaining love. We don't need to verbalize these thank you's all day long. Sometimes we can quietly adore Him. The Lord seeks worship that is sincere, and only worship that is sincere.

> The true worshipers will worship the Father in spirit and truth, for the Father is seeking such people to worship Him. *John 4:23 ESV*

CHAPTER 10   FRESH AIR TO THE SOUL

Like fresh air to the soul is the deep cleansing that follows conviction. Being washed by the Word feels good.

> When He (the Holy Spirit) comes, He will convict the world concerning sin.
>
> *John 16:8 ESV*

May we always be listening for this tender conviction recognizing the One who loved us enough to suffer in our place. It is He who wore the crown of thorns, it was He who endured the mocking of sinners against Himself to bring us into freedom as the beloved children of God.

It is by opening our hearts to the One who speaks to us so gently from Heaven, that we are cleansed.

> If we confess our sins, He is faithful and just to forgive us our sins and to cleanse us from all unrighteousness.   *1 John 1:8 ESV*

Conviction is a breath of fresh air. Breathe it in deep.

THE VALUE OF CONFESSION

> But the goal of our instruction is love from a pure heart and a good conscience and a sincere faith.
>
> *I Timothy 1:5 NAS*

God appreciates raw honesty. The absolute sincere confession of our sin opens the door to forgiveness and cleansing. We need to confess today and we need to confess every day. We need to confess every time anything comes in the way of our fellowship with God. And I need to confess that I need to confess more than I do. A sincere confession may sound like this:

"Dear Jesus. I'm bent out of shape and I'm worried. You know I eat too much. I believe in you. I am trusting in you. You are my only hope." You get a sense that He is saying, "Peace, my child. I've got this," and extends His hand to ours. Utter honesty is the only kind of prayer that God listens to. He loves us to humble ourselves and pray.

There are times when I need a little extra power to overcome; and I confess my sin to another believer. In order to get free of the filthiness hiding in the dark corners of my heart and to silence the guilt festering in my mind, I might need to have a frank talk with a Bible-believing fellow Christian.

James 5:16 ESV

Notice the Bible refers us to a nice one-another kind of confession—not a robed-clergy-behind-closed-doors kind of confession. It's a straight talk with another sincere believer just like us, someone who can feel what we are feeling, who understands our weakness, and who will pray for us in faith. The joy of confession is that when we bring our sin to the light, it becomes light.

When anything is exposed by the light, it becomes visible, for anything that becomes visible is light. *Ephesians 5:13 ESV*

Did you catch that? When you bring your sin to the light in Christ—when you confess the truth just as it is—it becomes light. The light of exposure to God's love purifies and cleanses you from all unrighteousness.

He is faithful not only to forgive, but also to cleanse us…completely!

As far as the east is from the west, so far does He remove our transgressions from us. As a father shows compassion to his children, so the Lord shows compassion to those who fear Him. For He knows our frame; He remembers that we are dust. *Psalm 103:10 ESV*

I CONFESS

> *St*olen waters are sweet, and bread
> eaten in secret is pleasant. But he knows
> not that the dead are there. *Prov. 9:17 KJV*

AGE 21. This is a story that is hard for me to tell. I never confessed it to anyone, and for that reason I am all the more ashamed to tell it now. But Christ has set me free from condemnation, and if I could, I would go back and confess to the people involved, and offer to pay for what I stole. The truth is, I stole food. As a young adult. And not just once. Regularly. And not because I was poor. I was well cared for. And I was a believer when I did it.

This happened at a lovely youth camp in Maine. I was a counselor, newly born again; and we ate dinner family style, counselors and campers together at a table. For me, eating at a table with younger people watching and other counselors too was torture. I would pass on seconds and take only small helpings to make sure everyone else at my table had enough. Dinner hour was short, and there never seemed to be enough time for me to get seconds on anything, yet I never spoke up. I would walk out of the mess hall as hungry, almost, as I walked in.

In back of the mess hall was the camping equipment shed, where individual boxes of sugared cereals were stored unopened in preparation for backpacking trips.   There I was drawn after dinner night after night, consuming box after box of sugary cereal, trying not to, wading in guilt even as I sought a way to justify my actions. Eventually I was caught, as you might expect, and I lied. I never told the truth. I said it had not been me who had been eating out of the shed. It must have been a raccoon.

But of course a raccoon could not unlock the shed, as I had. It was a sorry pitiful excuse, and I was a sorry excuse for a human being, much less a child of God.

> If we say we have no sin, we deceive
> ourselves, and the truth is not in us.
>> *I John 1:8 ESV*

But how could I confess that I was afraid to eat in front of people, that I didn't know how to eat, and I was just trying to be a good example? It all seemed so ludicrous, I was sure they would think I was crazy.

So now, though the camp is closed and the people long gone, if you can hear me Kris Ann and Hiawatha Camp staff, please accept my confession and apology. I would gladly reimburse what I stole seven times over.

NO REGRETS

There is a secret that Satan doesn't want you to know: if he can't terrorize you with regret… if he can't destroy your faith… if he can't get you back into a futile cycle of dieting, bingeing and guilt…Satan will give up and slink away.

You've heard Satan's voice. "You've really blown it this time. You might as well give up. Did you really think you could learn how to eat? You're hopeless." … And then, if you listen closely, you might hear his raucous laughter in the background. Satan is the one who condemns. God does not condemn.

The voice of God might convict though. He might let you see that you've been trusting in food when He alone can soothe your grief or satisfy your longing or enliven your day. If that is the case, humbly agree with God, ask Him to help you, and trust that He will. Healing will follow on the wings of your prayer.

Next time you hear that raspy voice of Satan trying to drag you into guilt, shut it down. Before he spits out another word, take up the sword of the Spirit and boldly quote the Word. "All things are lawful to him who believes." "Everything created by God is good." Whatever Scripture comes to your mind, affirm it and hold fast to the freedom you have in Christ. Then thank God for the food that you ate, and thank Him sincerely, asking the Lord to use it for His kingdom. Thank God for every single calorie. And you have won.

Submit yourselves therefore to God. Resist the devil, and he will flee from you.

James 4:6 ESV

Satan really is not as powerful as he would like us to think. The Bible tells of a day we'll see the devil and be amazed, saying,

Is this the man who made the earth tremble, who shook kingdoms?

Isaiah 14:16 NAS

And really, who is Satan to criticize the children of God?

It is God who justifies. Who is to condemn? Christ Jesus is the one who died—more than that, who was raised—who is at the right hand of God, who indeed is interceding for us. *Romans 8:31 ESV*

Let that Scripture root itself deeply in your heart. Soak up more and more Scriptures and you will find that overcoming condemnation becomes easier and easier. As your spiritual walls are built and strengthened by the Word of God, you will soon find the freedom that Christ promises. Satan will pack up and go home.

LET NO ONE JUDGE YOU...not even yourself

So what do you do if you're home and you have eaten eight times more than you think you really needed? The Bible is very clear—there is no condemnation for those who are in Christ Jesus.

> **There is now no condemnation for those who are in Christ Jesus.** *Romans 8:1 NIV*

Repeat:

> **There is now no condemnation for those who are in Christ Jesus.**

It's the truth. The price was paid at the cross. Out of His deep love for you, Christ took upon Himself every mess you have made in your life. You have been declared "not guilty" forever.

Now let's look at what you've just done. The Bible says the wisdom from above is peaceful, so let's stay peaceful. It also says that anything which is not done in faith is sin.

> **But he who doubts is condemned if he eats, because his eating is not from faith; and whatever is not from faith is sin.** *Romans 14:23 ESV*

But what if we're not sure if we sinned or not?

> **Therefore do not let anyone judge you by what you eat or drink** *Colossians 2:16 NIV*

Write that on your heart. You'll need it. "Let no man judge you in food or drink." That means nobody—not your mom, not your dad, nor your slim sister nor your health-nut mother-in-law. Not your boyfriend, not your doctor, not your yoga instructor, not the models in the magazines—nobody. And that includes YOU. You are likely your harshest critic. Don't look in that mirror and judge yourself. Don't judge yourself at all.

I used to look at myself and see imperfections (more specifically, flab) and believe that I had sinned against God. I was ashamed. Soon I'd be eating again, not out of hunger, but out of insecurity and rage—rage at myself for believing that I could be thin when it was perfectly obvious I could never be (or so I thought). What I didn't know is that the guilt was spawning the eating episodes, and the self-criticism was spawning the guilt. Judge nothing before the time, the Bible shouts again and again.

> **Judge nothing before the appointed time; wait until the Lord comes. He will bring to light what is hidden in darkness and will expose the motives of the heart.** *I Cor. 4:5 NIV*

Look in the mirror and say, "Interesting. This is what I look like now. Thank you God I am in your hands." The Bible does not tell us what we should look like. There is no weight chart in the Bible. Notice the Ten Commandments don't include a restriction on carbs, fat, alcohol, sugar or chocolate. The fact is, these are a shadow. Let us love one another, and let us love our bodies.

> **For no one ever hated his own flesh, but nourishes and cherishes it, just as Christ does the church.** *Ephesians 5:29 ESV*

Let's do that. Let's cherish our bodies. Let's be thankful for everything they are. And everything they will be:

> **The Lord Jesus Christ, who will transform our lowly body to be like His glorious body.** *Philippians 3:20 ESV*

We are a work in progress. His work. Believe and Know that He is teaching us how to eat. We don't need to weigh ourselves. I'd get rid of that nasty judge they call a scale. Throw it out. You know if you're healthy or not. You know if you are following God's Spirit. And if we fail, praise God. We will trust and obey. God is Good. He knows we are but dust. He knows we are weak. Paul showed us how to think about ourselves when he said, "I know of nothing against myself…"

> **But with me it is a very small thing that I should be judged by you or by any human court. In fact, I do not even judge myself. For I am not aware of anything against myself, but I am not thereby acquitted. It is the Lord who judges me.** *I Corinthians 4:3 ESV*

At the point you realize you just mindlessly consumed an entire box of graham crackers, that is the perfect time to thank God for what you ate. It's never too late to turn it over to Jesus, the lover of our souls.

I FEEL FAT (this too will pass)

It's one of those days. You were doing so well, but now you feel heavy. You ate too much. Or did you? Does the fact that you feel fat today mean that you have given in to lust?

No, it does not. We walk by faith, not by sight. Faith is not a feeling. The only way you can know if you are in sin is when God's Spirit convicts you. When our bodies seem to groan under their own weight, we can turn the feeling over to God and listen for His counsel, but we must not automatically conclude that we are in sin. Stomachs stretch when they are full. They shrink when they are empty. If they never stretched, they would only shrink and shrink and shrink until they disappeared. We can't rely on our own understanding, or on appearances.

Those days will come with less and less frequency as you abandon yourself to the leading of the Holy Spirit, but they will come. Those fat feelings are, like every other test we face, opportunities to strengthen our faith. Through them, we learn to choose Christ, choose Christ, choose Christ even when our feelings tell us we should do something foolish like diet.

We may feel that sluggish fat feeling when we're tired, worn out, and sleep deprived. We're likely to feel it when the food in our stomach is just sitting there stagnant. undigested, due to lack of exercise. There are times we'll feel uncomfortable with our bodies for any number of reasons, but there is still one and only one answer. Be honest with the Lord.

> **If any of you lacks wisdom, let him ask God, who gives generously to all without reproach, and it will be given him.**
>
> *James 1:6 ESV*

Remember when the prophet Samuel came to anoint God's chosen king? He almost chose the wrong guy. He looked at the tall, stately, oldest son and thought, "This must be the one," but God said no.

> **Do not look on his appearance or on the height of his stature, because I have rejected him. For the Lord sees not as man sees: man looks on the outward appearance, but the Lord looks on the heart.** *I Samuel 16:7 ESV*

Looking to Christ, willing to do His will, you can be confident that you are in His will no matter how much you eat. And you must hold on to that confidence.

> **Do not throw away your confidence, which has a great reward.** *Hebrews 10:35 ESV*

Strive to live in close communion with the Lord while you choose your food, while you prepare it, and while you eat it. And when you are done, give thanks. This trial will pass as soon as you have placed your absolute trust in God

Let the Holy Spirit lead and soon you will realize the potential you were made for. You will not hover endlessly around the cupboard or the refrigerator. You will find things to do and you will do them. You will find reserves of energy you never knew you had.

You must learn the secret of being full as well as the secret of being hungry.

> I have learned to be content in whatever circumstances I am... I have learned the secret of being filled and going hungry, both of having abundance and suffering need. *Philippians 4:11 NAS*

Both require faith. Both require looking to the Lord, looking to the Holy Spirit, and giving thanks. When I am full, I will lay my hand on my stomach, thank Him for the food I have eaten, asking Him to bless every calorie for His Kingdom.

The important test before God is not, "Did you eat or not eat?" The important test is, "Are you holding fast to Him right now?"

Remember, the Lord looks on the heart. As soon as your confidence is in Christ and Christ alone, the victory is won.

YES, THANK YOU LORD

So here it is. Don't assume that if you pick up a Hostess Twinkie you are a sinner. Maybe God just wants you to read the ingredients. Don't assume that looking in the cupboards an hour after Thanksgiving dinner means that you are a sinner. It might be that you need to see what groceries you will need. Or maybe there is something more you need to eat. The point is, if you are humbly submitted to God (which means letting Him lead) you can absolutely trust Him…and you must!

Moment by moment wait upon and listen to His still, small voice. To rush ahead in doubt is to sin.

> **Whoever has doubts is condemned if he eats, because the eating is not from faith. For whatever does not proceed from faith is sin.** *Romans 14:23 ESV*

So recognize this: eating more than we ever would have thought we should eat does not make us sinners. God knows the needs of your body, and He supplies us amply with all good things. He knows just the right combination of foods to make you sleek, slender, handsome, beautiful and wise.

Let's say you find yourself taking thirds and fourths, maybe sixths, and it's not even lunchtime. So what? If you are in God, looking to Him, then trust and eat! It happens to me all the time. "Dear God, this is a lot! Wow! Thanks! Too much! Wow! And this?! Thanks!

Gee, whiz, and you want me to eat that too?" That's the way it goes with you and the Heavenly Father. He saturates you in His love. He doesn't deprive.

There are times when the Holy Spirit has distracted me with something else to do when I kind of felt like eating, but most of the time I have been led to eat more frequently and more abundantly than I ever would have allowed myself based on my own mental perception of what to eat. Do you see the difference? God loves you. Your fleshly mind does not.

So, beloved, please don't avoid eating, thinking you are victorious. Depriving yourself now will only disrupt your body's optimum functioning, and will probably mean you will be stretching your stomach out later. Beloved, eat when you're led.

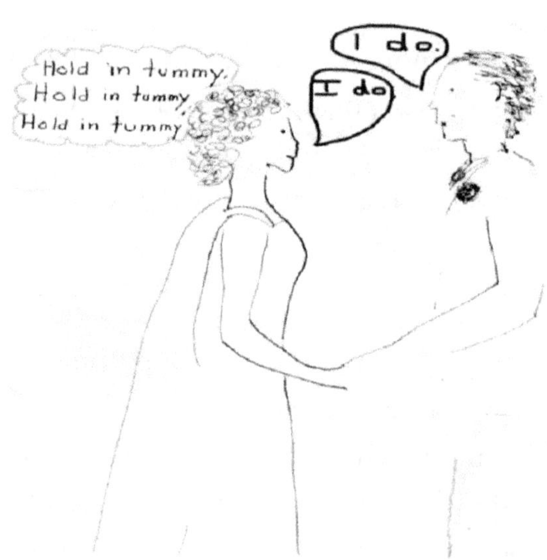

WHAT A JOY TO BE FREE

AGE 23. I never found out who gave us the plaque—a wedding present that hung on our wall through the most difficult years of my life—white letters printed on a light blue background, mounted on a block of stained wood:

> Thou wilt keep him in perfect peace,
> whose mind is stayed on thee:
> because he trusteth in thee.   Isaiah 26:3

The plaque was obviously second hand, probably from a thrift store, but that verse taught me how to endure years of suffering, and proved more valuable than any of the fancy tableware or silver we received.

LOVE SLAVES

Six of the epistles—Romans, Philippians, Titus, James, Jude and 2 Peter—begin with the authors referring to themselves as willing bondslaves of Christ. A bondslave is one who freely gives himself up to another's will. The apostles had settled in their hearts once and for all whom they served. They knew there are only two choices, and they rejoiced to be bondslaves of the One True God.

> No slave can serve two masters, for either he will hate the one and love the other, or he will be devoted to the one and despise the other. You cannot serve God and mammon.
>
> *Luke 16:13 ESV*

You know it too. We can't be led by the flesh and still serve God. We can't serve man's opinion and at the same time serve God. We can't be a servant to self will and still serve God. We can't conform ourselves to the fashion of the age and still serve God. No slave can serve two masters.

> Do you not know that if you present yourselves to anyone as obedient slaves, you are slaves of the one whom you obey, either of sin, which leads to death, or of obedience, which leads to righteousness?
>
> *Romans 6:15 ESV*

And here is the very good news:

> Thanks be to God, that you who were once slaves of sin have become obedient from the heart to the standard of teaching to which you were committed, and, having been set free from sin, have become slaves of righteousness. *Romans 6:15 ESV*

And we read again:

> "It is the Lord Christ to whom you are enslaved." *Colossians 3:24 ESV*

Why is this good news? Why is it good news to be a slave of Christ?

It is good news because the slave of Christ is free. To be a bondslave of Christ is to be led by the perfect and holy wisdom of God rather than by the blind dictates of the will. To be a slave of Christ—to put myself at His disposal every moment—is to experience the peace of riding on a cloud. To be His bondslave is to experience perfect love, incredible power, joy unspeakable. It is to be filled with the breath of the Almighty.

Jesus too abandoned His will to do that of the Father. He said:

> "I can do nothing on my own initiative." *John 5:30 NAS*

To be like Jesus, totally and completely subservient to the Father. This is freedom. There is no joy apart from this.

THE GREAT RELIEF

When I am in an urgent situation, when life seems to be coming down hard in all directions, I pray to God from my innermost Spirit. And it sounds like another language. When I am driving in the car, I enjoy singing in tongues. In the restroom and all through the day, I want to be praying in tongues. I love to pray and sing in tongues! Through it I am strengthened in amazing ways.

If you have not received the gift of tongues, I encourage you to seek this precious gift, and all the others. To pray with tongues is a holy release and you will be overwhelmed with the peace that floods your soul when you do.

> He that speaketh in an unknown tongue speaketh not unto men, but unto God: for no man understandeth him; howbeit in the spirit he speaketh mysteries. *I Cor. 14:1 ESV*

For most of the years of my Christ-following life, I was around no one else who believed in speaking in tongues, but I continued to do so because 1) it built me up in my faith, 2) it soothed me, 3) the Bible encourages it. Paul said:

> "I wish that you all spoke in tongues."
> *I Corinthians 14:5 NAS*

Some teach that tongues have ceased. They quote *1 Corinthians 12*, which does say that tongues will cease, but the very same verse says that knowledge will cease. Until knowledge ceases, we should not be teaching that tongues have ceased.

Some teach that the early church had a lot of trouble with disruptions in church, so it is better not to be involved with spiritual gifts. But Paul said,

> **I thank God that I speak in tongues more than all of you.** *I Corinthians 14:17 NIV*

True, the Bible says not all speak in tongues. *(I Corinthians 12)* But do you want to be built up in your faith? Paul says, **"He who speaks in a tongue edifies himself."** As our churches begin to function again in the power of the Spirit, with tongues, and interpretation of tongues, and prophesying, and gifts of healing and miracles, the world will be turned upside down for Christ.

Do you want the fullness of God? Press in, pray fervently, and ask God for this precious gift. I know people who received the gift of tongues alone in their rooms, after reading the scripture, believing and asking. Others have received the gift simply as they fervently sought God, without having ever known it existed.

Worship the Lord in spirit and truth, and as you draw in, at some point you will be amazed to hear what may seem like gibberish coming from your mouth! Keep your eyes fixed on Christ, letting your tongue praise Him in this new way, and you will understand the great relief that comes from worshipping God in the Spirit.

NO TIME FOR THE DEVIL

The devil wants to prevent you from being of value to the kingdom of God, and you don't have time to fuss with him. Instead:

> **Submit yourselves therefore to God. Resist the devil, and he will flee from you.**
> *James 4:7 ESV*

Notice the order: First, submit to God. Then resist the devil. The fact that you want to eat another piece of garlic bread does not mean the devil is around. Submit to God and see how He leads you. With your heart primed to do God's will and His alone, He will lead you safely past the garlic bread or to eat the garlic bread and either way there are no worries.

Standing up against the the devil and resisting demonic powers works especially well out loud. Verbalizing what you are saying amplifies what you believe. *(Romans 10:10, Mark 11:23, I John 1:9)*

So to resist the devil, speak the truth in confidence. "Jesus defeated Satan at the cross. Satan has no power over me. I am a child of the Most High God." Keep expressing in words what you know to be true, centering on the cross and the finished work of Jesus Christ until you know the devil has given up and fled. (He will. Satan hates to hear about the cross.) In fact, at the name of Jesus, demons tremble. *(James 2:19)*

TO FAST FOR RESULTS

Fasting won't teach you how to eat, but it can unlock strongholds that have kept you in bondage year after year. It can help you see unspiritual habits that preserve these strongholds, and show you, as Jesus said:

Life is more than food.   *Luke 12:23 ESV*

Fasting is for those who want to press in deeper, grow closer to the Lord, and be freed from worldly habits. Right fasting brings power. Going without food for a period, if it is led and initiated by God, can absolutely loose those bands of wickedness and lift off your shoulders the heavy burdens you carry. Early in my Spirit-led walk I undertook a fast to break the power of lust carried down for generations in my family. The fact that His grace was sufficient to carry me through six days of fasting leads me to believe it was God leading me, and I felt freer at the end.

But as Solomon said, "For everything there is a season." Wait for the Holy Spirit's breath to give you the leading and strength to fast. Don't try it out of self will. Remember the Pharisee who stood in the temple praying?

God, I thank You that I am not like other people: swindlers, unjust, adulterers, or even like this tax collector. I fast twice a week.....   *Luke 18:11 NAS*

What was Jesus's response to the Pharisees rigorous fasting? Jesus said that he did not go to his house justified, "For everyone who exalts himself will be humbled, but he who humbles himself will be exalted."

Wait a minute. Isn't fasting humbling yourself? Not for that Pharisee. Twice a week he fasted, but it was an act of pride, and God was not pleased.

We see then that asceticism, the practice of severe denial of physical needs for the sake of discipline, is not the way of our Loving Heavenly Father.

> If with Christ you died to the elemental spirits of the world, why, as if you were still alive in the world, do you submit to regulations— "Do not handle, Do not taste, Do not touch" (referring to things that all perish as they are used)— according to human precepts and teachings?
>
> These have indeed an appearance of wisdom in promoting self-made religion and asceticism and severity to the body, but they are of no value in stopping the indulgence of the flesh.
>
> *Colossians 2:20 ESV*

You heard it from Paul. Ascetism and severity to the body are of no value in curbing the flesh. Depriving yourself of food against the wishes of the Holy Spirit— who if you would let Him lead would guide you to eat— is not only foolish, it is dangerous. When we turn a deaf ear to the leading of the Holy Spirit, we set ourselves in opposition to God. We must abide in the vine, or whatever we do will only work against us.

As the Lord God leads through His Spirit, fasting is an incredibly helpful tool in the journey from food addiction to sane, sensible, eating habits. But it's not a way to lose weight. Keep that in mind. It is a chance to draw close to God and hear what He has to say. Walk in God's Spirit, eager to do His will, and whether He leads you to fast or not, you will find victory over lust and greed.

Walk by the Spirit, and you will not gratify the desires of the flesh. *Galatians 5:16 ESV*

TO FAST OR NOT TO FAST

Fasting is a blessing, but it's not the way to lose weight. In fact, God has designed us so that when we fast, our metabolism slows down and our body stores fat. That's a good thing if you're starving. It's a bad thing if you want to lose weight.

However, to fast under the leading of the Holy Spirit in order to break the bonds of wickedness that have held us captive…that is wise. To do so is to announce, as Jesus did, that your food is to do the will of your Father in Heaven.

> **"I have food to eat that you know not of…My food is to do the will of Him that sent me, and to finish His work."** *John 4:32 KJV*

To fast or not to fast? The answer is simple: Only if God leads. And you'll know it's a fast He has called, because it's relatively easy (His yoke is easy) as you surrender your will to Him. Looking to Christ as you go through your day, you'll find peace and satisfaction without food.

Nutritionists say the best time to begin and end a fast is after arising in the morning, whether you are fasting for one day or five days or ten. That is because your bowels are most active in the morning. As the Lord leads, eat fresh fruits (green smoothies are terrific) to cleanse your system before and after the fast. Drink plenty of water throughout. And keep your eyes focused on Christ.

Usually the hard part of fasting does not have much to do with hunger, but with habit. You have a routine every morning that includes food. You have a schedule that revolves around times of eating. Suddenly you have way too much time: and that's one of the wonderful things about fasting. You have more time, and (I think you'll find) more energy, because your body is not involved in the heavy work of digesting.

The other hard part of fasting is, of course, the enjoyment of eating that you miss—the enjoyment of tasting, the enjoyment of chewing, the enjoyment of camaraderie at meals. If you can get past those things, and you can, you will find that your stomach can go quite a long time without causing much of a fuss. There might be arduous moments, but crying out in faith, "Jesus, you are my bread!" will get you through.

The tendency of some is to skip a meal because we think it is honoring God to do so, but this form of self-directed abstinence has nothing to do with Christ. All going without is likely to do—unless God has led you to do so—is to clog up your metabolism and cause you to stuff yourself later.   God does not desire sacrifice.

> ### Behold, to obey is better than sacrifice.
> *I Samuel 15:22 ESV*

To obey is better than sacrifice. Hang on to that. We can't gain God's favor by dieting. God only wants us to humbly submit to Him, tuned in to His gentle Spirit, willing to follow His leading. Everything else will follow.

CHAPTER 12
TRUE RICHES

Can you imagine being offered all the world's riches at once?

> The devil took Him to a very high mountain and showed Him all the kingdoms of the world and their glory. And he said to Him, "All these I will give you, if you will fall down and worship me."
>
> *Matthew 4:8 ESV*

Jesus knew exactly how to respond.

> It is written, "'You shall worship the Lord your God and Him only shall you serve.'"

Jesus had a very good reason for rejecting Satan's offer. Jesus knew as the Son of God that He already possessed all things. And guess what? So do we!

> All things are yours, whether Paul or Apollos or Cephas or the world or life or death or the present or the future—all are yours, and you are Christ's, and Christ is God's.
>
> *I Corinthians 3:21 ESV*

That's a kick, isn't it—to know all things are yours? The world is yours, life is yours, death is yours, the present is yours, the future is yours. Wow, huh? Everything is yours in Christ. And you are Christ's. Hallelujah!!!

TEMPTATION: THROW IT OUT!

> Lead us not into temptation, but deliver us from evil.
>
> *Matthew 6:13 ESV*

One of the best ways to avoid temptation—besides not buying it in the first place—is to pick it up and throw it out.

Leftover candy? Pitch it! I hate waste too, but consider the alternative—waste can or waistline. At least in the garbage, it's a one-time affair. But if you eat it, you are only feeding the monster, stretching its boundaries, tantalizing the tongue to want more—a choice far more wasteful in the long run.

What to do with pink candy hearts and jelly beans? It's okay to throw them away. It is more wasteful to put stuff into your bodies that will turn your digestive system into an acidic invitation for colds and flu or worse.

> It is not good to eat much honey.
>
> *Proverbs 25:27 ESV*

The same with Christmas candy (tooth decay waiting to happen), unhealthy food you find in the back of your cupboards, and that big jug of cheese puffs you bought last week that you wish you hadn't. Compost it. Crush it. Pulverize it. Throw it out. But ask the Lord first, so you don't change your mind later and try to fish it out of the garbage. Let the precious Holy Spirit lead. God will supply.

BUT ALL FOODS ARE CLEAN

Now, wait a minute. Didn't Jesus say that all foods are clean? Yes, He did.

> "Do you not see that whatever goes into a person from outside cannot defile him, since it enters not his heart but his stomach, and is expelled?" (Thus He declared all foods clean.) *Mark 7:18 ESV*

And what about those other Scriptures that say no food is unclean in itself *(Romans 14-15),* and that all foods from the market can be eaten *(1 Corinthians 10:23-10:31)?* Doesn't God say everything is lawful as long as we give thanks?

Yes, you can be sure that at any point in time, if you need to eat something highly refined and processed, you can eat it in good faith, thanking God for it.

> For everything created by God is good, and nothing is to be rejected if it is received with thanksgiving, for it is made holy by the word of God and prayer. *I Timothy 4:4 ESV*

And God did make all things, so one could argue that even the artificial ingredients were made by Him. However, I doubt that you would want to eat the packaging, which—by the same reasoning—was also made by Him.

So it boils down to this:

<blockquote>

All things are lawful, but not all things are helpful.   *I Corinthians 10:23 ESV*

</blockquote>

All foods are lawful, but not all things are helpful. All foods are lawful, but not everything sold as food is even food. Check out some of the list of ingredients on that innocent-looking box of mashed potato flakes: sodium bisulfite, BHA, monoglycerides, sodium acid pyrophosphate, and more.

God loves you and He loves me, each of us, as His own body. And our bodies are temples of the Holy Spirit.

<blockquote>

No one ever hated his own flesh, but nourishes and cherishes it, just as Christ does the church, because we are members of His body.   *Ephesians 5:29 ESV*

</blockquote>

All things are lawful, and Christ has granted us absolute perfect liberty in Him. As we yield to the Holy Spirit, we naturally do what is right and good. We are drawn to eat exactly what will satisfy our bodies and optimize our health. Giving our moment-by-moment choices to the Lord God, we find ourselves rejoicing continually in His overwhelming goodness. We taste and see: Yes! Yes! Yes! the Lord is Good!

THE CURE FOR CRAVING

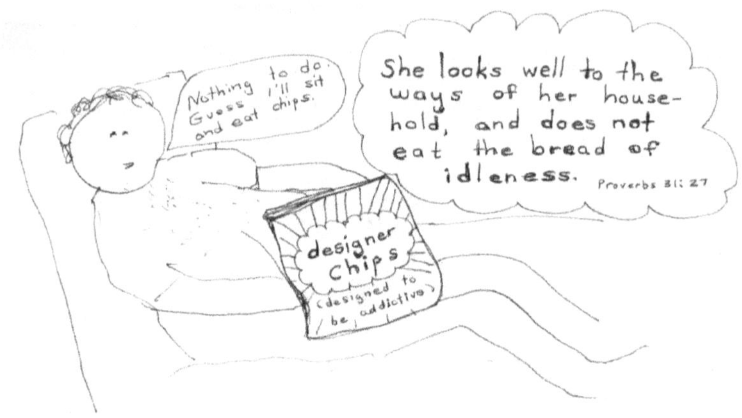

Before the Industrial Revolution few Americans were overweight. Why is it that they, who knew so little about nutrition, were slim; while we—with all knowledge at our fingertips, the exact calorie count of everything we eat and its precise nutritional content—are fat? The answer is pretty straightforward: They had plenty of hard physical work to do.

Hard physical work is a blessing. As a matter of fact, good hard work was part of the original paradise:

> **The Lord God took the man and put him in the Garden of Eden to work it and keep it.**
> *Genesis 2:15 ESV*

The Hebrew word translated here "work" is *abad* and is also translated "cultivate" and "plow." God intended for us to work. Why? because work feels good. It keeps our minds sharp and our bodies in tiptop shape. When we work hard, we sleep better:

> Sweet is the sleep of a laborer, whether
> he eats little or much, but the full stomach
> of the rich will not let him sleep.
>
> *Ecclesiastes 5:12 ESV*

Sweet, peaceful sleep is the reward of hard work.

Another wonderful blessing of work is that it drowns out the cravings.

> Slothfulness casts into a deep sleep, and
> an idle person will suffer hunger.
>
> *Proverbs 19:15 ESV*

Hard physical work keeps the appetite in check. But choose to plop down on the couch while the dishes are piled up, and within a few minutes you'll be itching for something salty or sweet. Ignore the call of household duties enough times and the unhealthy pounds magically appear. The Bible warned thousands of years ago of the unhealthy cravings induced by laziness.

> The craving of a sluggard will be the death
> of him, because his hands refuse to work.
>
> *Proverbs 21:25 ESV*

I understand laziness. For most of my young life I was the epitome of a sluggard (except for schoolwork). I lounged around, uncertain of what to do, unwilling to try my hand at anything. I was bored and listless and depressed. If only someone had shown me what to do and said, "Well, get busy."

There are times when maybe you're in a slump and you feel there is nothing to do but eat. It's a slow languishing feeling that envelops like a dark cloud, reducing your vision down to whatever you think might be tasty at the moment. You can fight through that by leaning entirely on the Lord's leading, moment by moment. He'll keep you busy, and even make it fun.

And too, the Bible mentions another cure for craving:

> **The craving of a sluggard will be the death of him, because his hands refuse to work. All day long he craves for more, but the righteous give without sparing.** *Prov 21:25 ESV*

Have you ever considered that giving might end the cravings? Our town holds a free community dinner once a week. An army of volunteers arrive, bringing a pot of soup, fresh bread, a salad. How satisfying it is for them to watch their food eaten by grateful folks.

Growing up, my family lived across the road from a poor family who, indications were, suffered from lack of food. Meanwhile, I suffered from too much food. How hard would it have been for me to get up off the couch and take something to them? How difficult would it have been to have opened my heart to my neighbor in need?

You crave. You are not alone. Craving is a universal temptation. Craving at its basic form is the idea that food is the solution for the way you are feeling now, and eating is the only thing to do when there is nothing else particularly worth doing. Yet, by the Spirit's guidance, we find joy in giving, joy in serving, joy in hard work.

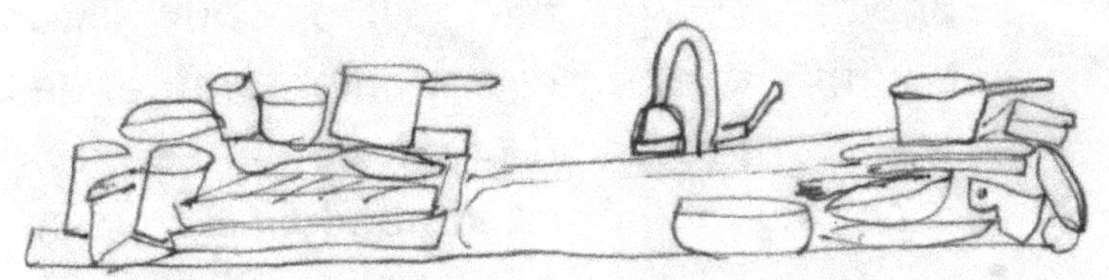

WHEN THE SPIRIT MOVES YOU

It bears repeating. How do we fill the time, if we don't fill it with food? God made us to be active. And the easiest way to be active is to work. Look what happened when Jesus's disciples were urging their master to eat.

> Jesus said to them, "My food is to do the will of Him who sent me and to accomplish His work. *John 4:34 ESV*

Work is food. Work is the antidote to craving. Solomon knew the value of work.

> The soul of the sluggard craves and gets nothing, while the soul of the diligent is richly supplied. *Proverbs 13:4 ESV*

If you find yourself drawn to lust, sucked into Satan's sewer system, let me ask you: How much of your day is involved in real work? Let's look at your house: does it glorify God, or is it falling apart before your eyes? How about your car? Your closets? Okay, maybe your own stuff is in order. How can you help somebody else? This is where joy is found.

Do we want the cravings to cease? Walk the elderly neighbors' dog. Offer to get her groceries. Wash her windows, visit the sick, spruce up a vacant lot, volunteer at the elementary school, shovel snow for a neighbor. Do some good old-fashioned work, and your body will actually need to eat, and you will be satisfied.

The excellent wife described in Proverbs 31 is an active woman, getting up early, preparing food for everybody, making clothes, even planting a vineyard. She doesn't eat the bread of idleness—that is, she doesn't eat just for something to do. The result of all this diligence?

The reason to keep moving is simple. God has created us to do so. It's not natural to sit on a couch or in a chair for hours at a time. Your body craves movement.

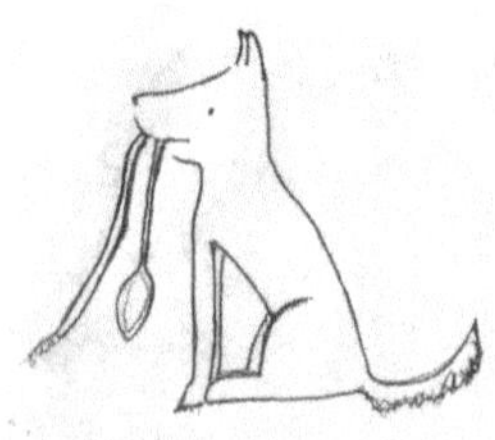

Can't get out? Stretch in every direction as far as you can. Why not? Anything you can do to step up your respiration and increase your blood flow will assist your body to do its job cleaning out waste from your blood stream… concurrently improving your mood. Draw in the oxygen of God.

We need stimulation. Our automatic tendency is to look for that stimulus in eating, but there are so many other ways. Our bodies were made for movement. Our hands were made for work. So if it's one of those days where you find yourself continually looking in the fridge and it seems no matter what you eat, you'll never be satisfied, take a moment. Stop. Listen to the Lord with an attitude of complete surrender. Wait, and you'll feel His gentle leading—not the harried "Do it now" or "Let's get this over with" of the will—but the gentle leading of the Holy Spirit of God who works in you.

For it is God who works in you, both to will and to work for His good pleasure.
Philippians 2:13 ESV

Stop and wait for the Lord. You'll be amazed what He leads you to do. It's always good. When that desire to be around food seems overwhelming, you might find He inspires you to cook something. Cooking is a creative act, best done in tune with God, and it is oh-so-helpful to know exactly what we are eating. Chopping vegetables, mixing liquids and solids, enjoying the textures, the sounds, the smells and colors of natural food connects you back to nature and satisfies your being in the way God intended.

God intended us to take time to enjoy our food, including its preparation. Cooking with the Holy Spirit satisfies. You will learn to appreciate and give thanks in a deeper way for all you have. Don't give up if you tried cooking and failed. No one has made more inedible flops than I have. But through those mistakes I am learning the principles of what makes food puff up, stick together, brown nicely, and taste good.

Even sewing is exercise, for both the body and mind. Scrubbing the floor is wonderful exercise, as is raking leaves, cleaning gutters, shampooing the carpet, washing the dog. It's all good. Find what you like. Like what you find. And sometimes shut yourself away and dance to the Lord. Your dance can be slow, balanced, and graceful; or fast, wild and jiggly. God loves it all.

Let them praise His name with dancing, making melody to Him with tambourine and lyre!
Psalm 139:3 ESV

Sing to the Lord in whatever funny voice you have. It is your heart tuned to His station that God adores.

THE LORD GIVES HIS BELOVED SLEEP

> It is in vain that you rise up early and go late to rest, eating the bread of anxious toil; for He gives to His beloved sleep.
>
> *Psalm 127:2 ESV*

One of Satan's favorite tactics is to wear down the saints through constant activity.

> He will speak out against the Most High and wear down the saints of the Highest One.
>
> *Daniel 7:25 NAS*

The enemy of your souls will try to induce you to do more good things, and more, and more! He'll try to convince you to wake up an hour earlier than usual so you can go running, then skip lunch and go for a walk, fast today and tomorrow, attend all the Bible studies and prayer meetings there are, volunteer at every church function, and finally, to pray on your knees for hours before going to bed.

God is much kinder than most of us think:

> It is in vain that you rise up early and go late to rest, eating the bread of anxious toil; for He gives to His beloved sleep.
>
> *Psalm 127:2 ESV*

Those activities could all be good, but if they overload you with anxious toil, you are depriving yourself of the blessed peace God offers, and missing out on the lovely quiet time with God we call "sleep."

The amount of sleep you get seriously affects your disposition. The amount of sleep you get directly affects the intensity and frequency of your urges to eat. Ghrelin is the hormone that alerts your mind that the body needs something to eat. When you are sleep-deprived, ghrelin are released all over the place yelling "Let's eat NOW!" However, after a good night's sleep, you won't hear a peep out of them until it's time.

And check this out. Leptin is the hormone that tells your body, "No more food needed now, thanks." When you get enough sleep, your leptin buddies are released. When you're sleep-deprived, leptin stay in hiding.

So good wholesome sleep quiets the "I'm hungry" hormones and releases the "Everything's fine" hormones. Why waste time staying up late? The news will get along without you. Perfectly clean house? Not important. Working too many hours at the job will just make your coworkers jealous.

Better is a handful of quietness than two hands full of toil and a striving after wind.

Ecclesiastes 4:6 ESV

Yes, come to think of it. It's time for bed.

THOU SHALT NOT WORSHIP.... DOCTORS

Should we run to the medicine chest? Or should we call the doctor first? Oh… wait a minute. Maybe we should look to the Lord first.

Yes. Why do we automatically look for healing from those who can not cure, people who can at best only remove symptoms? It is the Lord who heals.

> **Bless the Lord, O my soul, and forget not all His benefits, who forgives all your iniquity, who heals all your diseases.**
>
> *Psalm 103:2 ESV*

Heals all your diseases. Did you hear that? Oh, yes, and He will, if we will seek Him. That is not to say that He does not use doctors. He does of course. But your first choice should always and forever be the great Physician, I don't care how good your insurance is.

He who created every cell in our body and maintains its function is infinitely and absolutely capable of healing us—and why would He not? God is altogether love. Does He not wish to heal you? Jesus healed everyone who came to Him. Abandon unbelief. Ask in faith, and trust. He will do just as you asked… and way better.

> **Now to Him who is able to do far more abundantly than all that we ask or think,**

> according to the power at work within us, to Him be glory.
>
> *Ephesians 3:20 ESV*

Thank Him for the healing He will do before it has begun to emerge. Trust Him and trust Him and you will find that all the aches and pains you thought were just part of getting older will vanish. Seek and seek and you will find that severe troubles that have hung on so long will disappear as He opens your eyes to the cure.

Again, it boils down to being led by the Spirit. God is faithful and eager to clue you in to the problem if you harken to Him. Open your ears to Him before you ever seek another physician. Natural God-given healing remedies abound, and it is God's pleasure to lead us to the right answer as we seek knowledge.

So often the Holy Spirit has awakened my understanding to the cause of whatever pain I am experiencing. Sometimes He whispers to me a clue, and sometimes He leads me in a search online for natural (God-given) healing methods. It always leads to an aha! moment, which leads to a simple lifestyle change, and then to complete and total healing. I've not taken any medicine except a couple aspirin in a decade. Nor have I needed to. Bless the Lord.

Yes, I am thankful for doctors, but the Lord is my primary care physician.

THE GREAT PHYSICIAN

AGE 38: There was a time when severe headaches overwhelmed me again and again, forcing me to to seek the Lord more than I had ever sought Him before. Then came the day the pain was so excruciating, so unbearable, I would gladly have died rather than endure another moment. I cried out to Him with every ounce of my being, and the pain subsided to tolerable.

The next morning when I felt the pressure in my head returning, I determined to look to the Lord in real faith, choosing to believe without doubting that He could do what He said He could and He would.

And He did. I was led to the bathroom where the Holy Spirit drew my attention to a pink plastic syringe in the medicine chest I hadn't taken much notice of before. It had always just been there. The thought came to me to give myself an enema.

I had never done anything like that before, but I was constipated (my norm since childhood) so I investigated the idea. I wasn't even sure how to do it, but I squeezed the warm water into my rear end, and when a hard clod or two came out, the pain in my head vanished instantly. The next time my head began to feel twisted in knots, I did the same. Each time, eliminating the clogs in my colon instantly eliminated the pain in my head. The Lord had shown me I could solve the headache problem by solving the constipation problem! Bless the Lord!!!

But how could I stop being constipated? I really didn't want to continue with this routine for the rest of my life. I thought maybe drinking more water would help relieve it, but no matter how much I drank, it didn't seem to free up my digestion. I was still stuck most of the time.

I began seriously praying about it, calling out to Jesus, knowing He was listening, knowing He had an answer. I decided to take Him at His Word:

> I tell you, whatever you ask in prayer, believe that you have received it, and it will be yours.
>
> *Mark 11:24 ESV*

"Okay, Lord. I want to believe that I have already received the answer, but it's hard you know when I'm still clogged. I'm really uncomfortable, but I'm willing to believe." I'm talking to the Lord this way while shopping at the food coop, and suddenly I have the faith to believe His word is true. I will be healed.

At that moment I am led to a wooden shelf in the middle of the store where a little slip of paper is attached with a thumb tack. In tiny brown print is information on how to relieve constipation naturally! You can bet my eyes never left that piece of paper until I read it through again and again and memorized the main points.

I learned that day that undigested food, decomposing in your digestive system, sends toxins throughout the body, causing headaches and other problems. To keep your metabolism moving, the author advised four things, which I have never forgotten: fiber, sleep, water, and exercise. Fiber, sleep, water, and exercise.

So I had to think. I was eating a lot of fiber. I made our own whole grain bread, and we ate raw oats and sunflower seeds for breakfast. The problem was not lack of fiber. Sleep? I could use more, but the seven hours I got seemed to be adequate for now. Water? I was drinking plenty of that. Exercise? Oh…. I hadn't done much of that in ages. Taking care of kids was the extent of my exercise plan, and as they grew more independent there was less lifting and bending and stooping and holding, so yes, I knew that must be the missing ingredient in my life.

The next evening, I set out down the quiet country road we lived on, walking a few feet, jogging a few feet, walking, jogging, and made it as far as the next door neighbor's house where I turned around and came back. Nothing to brag about, but for me it was a breakthrough. I continued this routine every evening and soon I could jog most of the way, and I was feeling pretty good. What's more, after giving birth to four children, I felt my flabby uterus tuck back into place as my pelvic floor was strengthened. Best of all, I was free: No more constipation! I was alive again, it seemed, as I had not been alive in so long.

Oh, the exercise felt good, and oh, how good it felt to relieve myself the way God intended daily. Since that day (except for a couple times I have been exposed to toxic chemicals) I have never had another headache.

What I learned is that God sometimes lets us persist in our sickness so that we can be well. That may seem like a contradiction. It is just testimony to His mysterious wisdom. It would not glorify God for you to be healed and then require healing again the next day and every week thereafter. So our loving Heavenly Father in His omniscient mercy, allows us to be sick, all the while leading us to wholeness.

He will bend over backwards to help us find the source and cure of our sicknesses, if we will listen and believe the voice of the Holy Spirit.

The Lord may whisper to you to go to the doctor, and if so of course you should go, but more often He will have a solution for you right at your fingertips...some simple and straightforward lifestyle change that will make a world of difference in your health.

> He said to me, "My grace is sufficient for you, for My power is made perfect in weakness." *II Corinthians 12:7 ESV*

THOU SHALT NOT WORSHIP EXERCISE

> For physical training is of some value, but godliness has value for all things, holding promise for both the present life and the life to come.
>
> *I Timothy 4:8 ESV*

AGE 40. I was born again, baptized in the Spirit, knowledgeable of the Word... but I still worshipped idols. Although I did not realize it at the time, I worshipped the gods of beauty and thinness and now... I worshipped exercise. Vanity. Vanity.

I knew the first commandment of the Lord: "You shall have no other gods before Me" (Exodus 20:2), but I am ashamed to admit that a slim trim body was more important to me than the will of God. Every day I sought out alone time with Jesus by jogging many miles, but in actual fact I ran because I was afraid to be still. It was the fear of getting fat that made me run. My intense desire for a body without a trace of plumpness kept me from seeking God's will for me. And so I ran.

In the winter when I could not run I cross-country skied, a wonderful thing except when it controls you. One evening I was so desperate to exercise, so desperate to be model-thin, that after dinner I headed out alone on the trails. Pitch dark, another skier emerged out of nowhere and knocked into me. Her pole narrowly missed my eye, and gouged out a deep wound just below, leaving a scar on my face that was visible for years after. You'd think I would learn something from that.

But I didn't. The next season found me exercising my life away again in the vain attempt to be beautiful. I swam. Swimming is a wonderful sport, and I recommend it, as the Lord leads. But I didn't care if the Lord led me or not. I swam. Day after day I swam 36 laps at the Y, over and over, back and forth, ignoring my children and boring myself to death with the nothingness of it all, striving for my body to be sleek and beautiful. And I always felt I should be doing more. More exercise. More lengths. More striving.

Well, in the process, I gained big dark circles under my eyes from too-tight goggles. Eventually those ugly dark circles awakened me to the truth that seeking beauty or anything apart from the continual guidance of God's Holy Spirit is an offense to Him. I had sought for beauty instead of God, and ended up disfiguring my face in the process.

Those dark circles and that scar under my eye remained for many years, a visible testimony and reminder of my idolatry.

Oh, may I always remember to set my eyes on Christ.

THOU SHALT NOT WORSHIP
Someone Else's Body

Idols. They are not always carved statues. Sometimes they are the images carved in our minds.

> You shall not make for yourself a carved image...You shall not bow down to them or serve them.
> *Exodus 20:4 ESV*

Have you ever considered that that image in your mind—that image of what you should look like in a swimsuit—is an idol? If that thought rules your decisions, that image is an idol. Destroy it. Cast it off the pedestal of your mind and let it shatter below. Your body type, your body shape, your body size, belongs to God.

We won't realize His victory unless our goal is more love, more peace, more Jesus in our lives. The fact is, and this is a hard saying: We must be willing to be fat for Christ. Or thin. Whatever is His will for us. We don't know His perfect plan for our body.

What is considered the ideal body weight for a woman in some localities is a hefty fifty pounds greater than what is considered the ideal body weight for a woman of identical height elsewhere. Some countries, like Tonga, Mauritania and Nigeria, consider plumpness a blessing. And why not?

And for us as Christian believers? We have died, remember? Dead people don't worry about their weight.

> **For the death He died He died to sin, once for all, but the life He lives He lives to God. So you also must consider yourselves dead to sin and alive to God in Christ Jesus.** *Romans 6:8 ESV*

There's no need to compare our body to any one else's.

> **They measuring themselves by themselves, and comparing themselves among themselves, are not wise.** *2 Cor. 10:12 ESV*

Instead of focusing on my weight or my appearance, I have learned to focus on health. Am I healthy? What parts of my body are healthy? The ones that are not, I ask the Lord to fix. And He does! Looking at me, some might think I'm too thin. And some might think I'm too fat. I feel fine. Great, even. And I dare not judge by appearance that which God has done in me.

> **For they loved praise from men more than praise from God.** *John 12:43 NIV*

I give my body to you, Lord. Thank you for making me into your image. When I stand in front of the mirror, Jesus, help me to see it the way you do.

ON STAYING HUMBLE

The truth is, Satan doesn't care what you eat. What you eat will eventually be pooped out. *(Mark 7:19)* What Satan wants is your mind. And one of Satan's favorite ploys is to get you to judge your neighbor. If he can get you to look down on somebody else, that's enough to keep you from experiencing the love of God, the fellowship of the Holy Spirit, and the unity of the Body of Christ. The Scriptures warn us against trotting around with an air of superiority.

AGE 45. I was getting into exercise. First I ran a couple blocks, and then a few miles, and eventually got into triathlons where I won a few ribbons for my age group. I was pretty impressed with my own ability to stay slim.

During this time, I remember seeing my friend in bulging bicycle shorts, and thinking smugly, "Too bad for her. No self-control." Then, sure enough, my thighs would begin to bulge out like hers, even though it didn't seem like I was eating more. And I was exercising for hours every day! "What's going on here?" I wondered. Gradually, it dawned on me:

> Pride goes before destruction, and a haughty spirit before a fall.
>
> *Proverbs 16:18 ESV*

That was me. Haughty.

The next time I saw my friend in her bike shorts, I was a lot more compassionate and understanding. I guess that's the purpose for suffering in our lives, to increase our love for God and for one another.

But I didn't learn quickly. I continued to look down on anyone who wasn't slim and trim and fit, and at the same time found myself never quite slim, never quite trim, and never quite fit. Like the Pharisee in the temple, I would pray, "I thank thee God that I am not like other people: obese and out of shape. I exercise daily, drink only water, and eat only health foods." It never occurred to me that God would not approve.

And my weight began to climb. I was doing everything right, wasn't I? The ridiculousness of my struggle to lose weight while exercising myself to death finally drove me to humble myself and seek answers....at which point it again dawned on me that the current root of my struggles with food was pride.

It was as if Jesus was saying to me, "Why do you see the roll of fat that hangs over your sister's belt, but don't see the mountain of fat in your own heart? Or how can you say to your sister, 'You better lose a few pounds,' and not see the heavy load of pride you carry?"

I stood condemned. Thank God for the cross. Thank God for forgiveness and mercy. I need it again and again and again.

Jesus spoke this again to my heart:

> Judge not, that you be not judged. For with the judgment you pronounce you will be judged, and with the measure you use it will be measured to you.   *Matthew 7:1 ESV*

The same measure that I use to measure others will be used to measure me! Yikes!

> You have no excuse, O man, every one of you who judges. For in passing judgment on another you condemn yourself, because you, the judge, practice the very same things.   *Romans 2:1 ESV*

Well, eventually it dawned on me: I can pray for people who are struggling with food—the large lady at the grocery store, the obese man in the wheelchair, the children who suffer with too much food, and for my friend. I will bless them, and pray for their health.

So... I'm learning. God resists the proud. He gives grace to the humble.

OOPS

You think you've finally got it together. You're losing weight, feeling fine, and what you're doing seems to be working. You're feeling proud. Your clothes fit. You are telling people how it happened. "Yea, I've been drinking more water.... "I joined a speed walking class.... "I started never eating after 6:00 p.m.". Maybe it's eating raw vegetables, or starting every day with a fruit smoothie, whatever. It works for awhile, and it's wonderful! You feel great and you think you have the answer. Then, after you've told all of your coworkers about the new method, all of a sudden it doesn't work. You thought you had it figured out, and wham... it disappoints you… as always.

> **Therefore let anyone who thinks that he stands take heed lest he fall.** *1 Cor 10:12 ESV*

Remember where your weight loss came from. Was it by your own efforts, or was it by letting the Lord lead?

Take heart again. Though diets fail, methods disappoint, and every scheme falters, whoever places their hope entirely in the Lord will never be disappointed.

> **"Whoever believes in Him will not be disappointed.** *Romans 10:11 NAS*

The world would have you put your hope in something new—a new diet, a nutrition drink, an exercise program, whatever they are hawking. And your own brain will try to sell you ideas that may be fine in and of themselves, but they will not free you from the confusion and turmoil of what to eat and when.

There were so many times, thinking I had finally achieved the answer to keeping my body trim, the end was disappointment: whether it was swimming or drinking more fluids or yoga or giving up meat or eating less fat or eating more fat or running. Nothing, absolutely nothing, proved to be the real answer. Christ requires a deeper sacrifice, not only of the flesh but of the heart. He says to give up the rights to every ounce of our being, and we'll be free. It's true.

> **For whoever would save his life will lose it, but whoever loses his life for My sake will find it.** *Matthew 16:25 ESV*

So now remember when you have found relief from the cravings, when you are satisfied, when your body is trim and fit, remember that the solution was not in the natural food you were led to eat. The solution was not in the exercise God enabled you to undertake. The solution was not in the extra hour of sleep or the time spent outdoors. The solution was in dying—your willingness to die, that Christ might live through you.

Remember every time your brain comes up with a new plan: Jesus is our wisdom, our counsel, our hope, our transformation, our victory. The Holy Spirit is our guide. Halleluiah, Lord God Almighty!

TO KNOW THE LOVE OF GOD

For so long we ate to try to fill the hole in our heart that only the love of God could fill.

But how can we know God's love? How can we fill those empty spaces that yearn for love? Well, Jesus said:

> **For this reason the Father loves me, because I lay down my life.**   *John 10:12 ESV*

Did I read that right? Did Jesus say He was loved by God because He was willing to lay down his life? Yes, you bet He did. And we find love the same way.

> **What great love the Father has lavished on us, that we should be called children of God!**   *I John 3:1 NIV*

God loves us. He is devoted to loving us. It is Satan who blinds us to the love of God. It is Satan who muddles Christians' minds to prevent them from knowing they are loved. We see God's love poured out through Jesus, through His willingness to suffer for us, through His forgiveness, through every deliverance, every healing, every provision, every joy, every blessing, every tender miracle, every whisper from nature, every whisper from His Word, through life and faith and breath…the love of God poured out for you and me day after day moment by moment.

And finally, I am beginning to understand this great truth: To the extent that we believe the love of God, we experience the love of God. It's so very simple. To the extent that we believe the love of God, we experience His love.

Here and now I confess that I will no longer believe that God is not interested, or mad, or too far away. If a thought comes to bring on discouragement or dejection or any such thing I will recognize it as a lie, and will testify of the truth.

I hereby testify to myself and to the powers in heaven: God loves me perfectly, unconditionally, completely. I am loved with everlasting love! Jesus is preparing a mansion for me in eternity. I am His chosen bride.

With the same love that God the Father loves His Son, so I am loved. Jesus said so Himself:

> **As the Father has loved Me,
> so have I loved you.** *John 15:9 ESV*

Jesus calls us to abide, stay, and remain, in His love.